Copyright © 2024

First Edition

Page Contents

Page Contents

The Forgotten Herbal Treasures Book

Page Contents

Notice of Disclaimer

This book aims to provide information on natural medicines, cures, and remedies historically used by people. The publisher, editor, and authors present this information with the understanding that they do not offer any legal or medical advice. If you are ill, always consult your physician or a medical specialist.

This book does not claim to be comprehensive and does not include all available information on natural remedies. Despite the authors', editor's, and publisher's efforts to compile an accurate and useful collection of healing plants and remedies in North America, typographical and content errors may exist.

Therefore, this book should not be used as a medical guide. The authors, editor, and publisher accept no liability or responsibility for any loss or injury, direct or indirect, resulting from using the information in this book. It is your responsibility to consult your physician before using any potion, tincture, decoction, or other remedies from this book.

Some remedies and cures mentioned may not comply with FDA guidelines. The information in this book has not been reviewed, tested, or approved by any official testing body or government agency. The authors and editor make no guarantees, expressed or implied, about the results obtained from applying the information found in this book. Using any products described is at your own risk.

The authors, editor, and publisher hold no responsibility for the misuse or misidentification of plants using the contents of this book, or any health consequences for you or others. Some names and identifying details have been changed to protect privacy.

The Forgotten Herbal Treasures Book

Extracting the Beneficial Properties of Plants for Healing

Introduction

In the grand tapestry of human history, modern medicine emerges as a relatively recent addition. Its lineage pales in comparison to the enduring legacy of traditional healing practices. For millennia, humanity has relied on natural remedies, harnessing the medicinal gifts bestowed by nature. Despite the advent of scientific advancements, the age-old efficacy of herbal medicines endures unchanged. Regrettably, the wisdom surrounding these botanical remedies has waned over time. It is our aspiration that this tome serves as a beacon to revive and transmit this vanishing lore.

Herbal medicine often encounters skepticism from the pharmaceutical realm, yet it stands as the progenitor of much contemporary medical science. Many of today's pharmaceuticals seek to emulate the therapeutic bounty of nature. Yet, in the pursuit of patentable formulations, synthetic alterations become requisite, often yielding compounds laden with adverse effects. While modern and herbal medicine can coexist harmoniously, the latter offers a compelling alternative, often boasting lower costs and reduced risks—both to our finances and our well-being.

In a hypothetical world stripped of modern conveniences, herbal medicines may emerge as our sole recourse. Should the intricate web of manufacturing and distribution unravel, our reliance would pivot to locally cultivated remedies. Already, those versed in the art of herbalism tend to the earth, cultivating and transforming botanical treasures into potent elixirs of healing.

Embracing the cultivation and utilization of one's herbs confers several advantages over procuring supplements from commercial vendors. By nurturing and harvesting herbs firsthand, one ensures freshness and purity. The immediacy of preparation often enhances their potency, while the transparency of their origins instills confidence. Each herbal concoction crafted embodies purity, free from additives or adulterants, containing only the desired botanical constituents.

Guidelines for Gathering Herbs

All remedies derived from botanical sources originate as living organisms. These resources encompass more than the traditional concept of herbs, extending to trees, blossoms, underground structures, fungi, lichens, and beyond. While enthusiasts of herbal medicine often cultivate their own herb gardens, certain remedies are sourced from wild plants. Acquiring the skill to discern medicinal plants in their natural habitats is invaluable.

When utilizing visual aids for plant recognition, it's imperative to seek out images that portray plants across various stages of their life cycles. A comprehensive plant identification manual tailored to your geographical region is indispensable. While many individuals can identify plants when they're in bloom, their recognition falters outside of the flowering period. Given the brevity of most plants' flowering seasons, this limitation underscores the necessity for a broader understanding of botanical identification.

The time available for harvesting plants is often limited, especially considering the narrow window of opportunity during their flowering seasons. Prior to embarking on the harvesting process, it's crucial to ascertain how the herb will be utilized, specifically identifying which part of the plant holds medicinal value. It's unwise to assume uniformity in chemical composition throughout the entire plant. Frequently, medicinal properties are concentrated in the leaves or flowers, while in other cases, the bark or root may contain the desired compounds.

Optimal harvesting conditions typically entail gathering herbs early in the day, after the dissipation of dew but before the sun's heat evaporates essential oils. Whenever feasible, refrain from uprooting the entire plant, unless it's necessary for specific species. When harvesting leaves, it's customary to trim small branches, facilitating the drying process. For flowers, harvesting should occur promptly upon full bloom. In the case of seed collection, wait until the seeds reach maturity and the seed pod desiccates on the stem before harvesting.

Detailed harvesting instructions are provided for nearly every herb in this guide. When harvesting stems, such as with stinging nettle, ensure to leave a sufficient portion of the leafy stem intact, preserving the plant's vitality.

Cutting should be done just above the point where the leaves emerge. With certain plants like basil, substantial pruning—up to one-third of its original size—can be tolerated without fatal consequences. Responsible harvesting practices dictate the replenishment of wild resources through reseeding, replanting, and conscientious stewardship. Ethical harvesting demands meticulousness and reverence for the natural world.

A Step by Step Drying Herbs

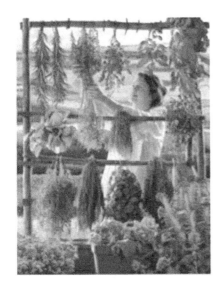

Traditionally, herbs are dried naturally without the aid of additional heat sources. Bundling them together by tying their stems with string or rubber bands, then hanging them in a warm, dry location, is a common practice. Hanging them upside-down by their bundled stems facilitates the drying process. For those drying larger quantities or doing so regularly, drying racks are an option. However, makeshift methods like hanging them from a coat hanger, a nail on the wall, or a curtain rod over a window yield similar results. Alternatively, spreading flowers or leaves on a cookie sheet or pizza pan allows for effective drying.

When collecting seeds, securing a paper bag over the bundled stems catches the seeds as the pods dry and release them. The duration of drying can vary, taking up to three weeks depending on the plant and its moisture content. For herbs with slow drying rates, like rosemary, it's preferable to strip the leaves off the stems and spread them on a drying rack to expedite the process, as the leaf coating can retain moisture. Ensure the herbs are fully dry before storage.

While using a dehydrator with temperature control is an option, it's essential to maintain a low temperature to prevent scorching or burning. Regular monitoring is crucial to prevent over-drying. Once dried, separate the leaves from the stems. Smaller leaves can be easily removed by lightly pinching the stem between your thumb and forefinger and running it down from top to bottom. Larger leaves with thicker stems may require individual cutting or pinching, removing them as close to the leaf as possible.

Store the dried herbs in sealed glass jars until ready for use. This ensures their preservation and maintains their potency.

Steps for Encapsulating Powdered Herbs

If you visit a health food store for herbs, you'll often find them available in powdered form, encapsulated for convenience. This method is particularly advantageous when administering herbs to individuals unaccustomed to herbal remedies. There are two primary approaches to encapsulating herbs, but before that, you need to grind the herbs into a powder. This can be achieved by using a food processor, electric coffee mill, or, for a more traditional method or during power outages, a mortar and pestle.

For herbal blends, a scale is necessary to measure out the various herbs accurately. It's crucial to thoroughly mix the powdered herbs to ensure uniform concentration in each capsule. Capsules are available in three sizes: "0," "00," and "000," and they can be filled manually or with the assistance of a filling machine.

The manual method involves placing the powder in an oversized bowl and individually opening the capsules by hand. The powder is then scooped into both sides of the capsule and compressed as the capsule is closed

Capsule filling machines offer a more efficient option. These machines come

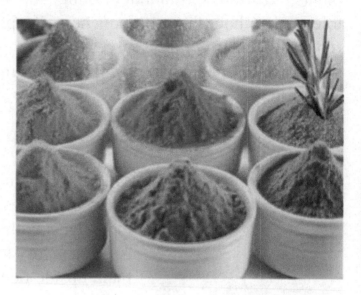

sizes to match the capsules being used and consist of plates with holes to hold the capsule halves and a base. Capsules are separated, with the thinner, longer part placed in the base plate. A funnel is used to fill the plate with capsule halves, which then fall into the holes. The same process is repeated for the top plate.

To fill the capsules, the powdered herbs are poured onto the bottom plate and distributed using a scraper. Any excess powder is removed before closing the capsules by aligning the top and bottom plates and pressing down multiple times.

While effective, capsule filling can be tedious and time-consuming. Having company or assistance during the process can make it more bearable. Once filled, the capsules are stored in jars for future use.

Creating Herbal Water Infusions: Cold and Hot Approaches

Tea and coffee, quintessentially, embody the concept of infusion, typically enjoyed piping hot. However, their chilled counterparts often undergo a similar process, initially infused with heat before cooling. Yet, it's entirely feasible to cold-infuse them, albeit with a slower pace. Patience becomes a virtue in this cold-infusion journey. Here, the essence of herbs effortlessly melds with water, a process replicable across various botanicals. Traditionally, herbs find their way into hot infusions as teas, either singularly or in harmonious blends tailored to specific wellness needs.

The allure of hot infusion lies in its prowess to extract a bounty of essential constituents from plant tissues. Heat, with its gentle coercion, dismantles cell barriers, fortifying the infusion's potency. However, the warmth of hot infusion may also coax out unwanted elements, such as bitterness, tainting the brew.

In such instances, the cool embrace of a cold infusion proves advantageous. Certain herbs, particularly those endowed with mucilaginous properties, thrive in a cold extraction environment, preserving their innate virtues.

Lemon balm, marshmallow, slippery elm, and comfrey stand as testament to the efficacy of cold infusion.

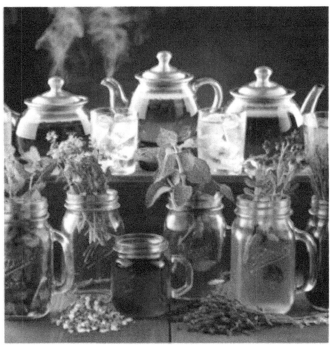

Enter sun tea, perhaps the pinnacle of cold infusion craft. Loose herbs, left to dance freely or nestled within a cheesecloth, grace the vessel, awaiting their transformation. Dosage remains simple: a teaspoon or two of dried herb per eight ounces of water. Prior to their icy immersion, dried herbs receive a gentle moistening, while their fresh counterparts require no such preparation. Awaiting a minimum of 48 hours, the cold infusion gradually coaxes forth the herbs' treasures, a testament to patience rewarded and wellness embraced.

Tea

Herbal tea stands as a ubiquitous conduit for harnessing the medicinal potential of herbs. As previously noted, it represents a prime example of a "hot infusion," excels in drawing out the advantageous constituents from a myriad of herbs. Unlike cold infusions, which demand patience due to their lengthier process, hot infusions yield results within mere minutes. The versatility of herbal tea extends to the choice between fresh and dried herbs, each imparting its distinct profile to the brew. It's essential to recognize that the reaction of each herb varies depending on its moisture content, prompting the need to adhere to specific recommendations tailored to the herb or herbal blend in question. This ensures the optimal extraction of beneficial properties and enhances the therapeutic potential of the herbal tea.

Decoctions

A decoction serves as a potent rendition of a hot infusion or tea, particularly beneficial for herbs that are reluctant to release their therapeutic compounds, or for tougher components like roots or woody parts. It's also an ideal method for creating a concentrated herbal supplement, especially suitable for individuals such as children, animals, or those who may not consume sufficient quantities of a standard hot infusion to derive its benefits.

To craft a decoction, begin with cold distilled or purified water. The cold temperature is crucial for maximizing the extraction of nutrients from the herbs. Opt for an earthenware, glass, or glazed ceramic pot to avoid any undesirable reactions with metallic vessels, which could affect the final flavor.

Maintain a ratio of 1 ounce (28g) of dried herbs per 16 ounces (500ml) of water. Decoctions are typically prepared in quantities meant for immediate or short-term consumption, as they do not retain freshness beyond a few days in the refrigerator. For longer storage, tightly seal the decoction or freeze it (ice cube trays are convenient for this purpose). Adding two tablespoons of alcohol (like vodka, rum, or brandy) per cup (8oz) enhances preservation.

Here's a step-by-step guide to creating a decoction:

Prepare the herbs by crushing, chopping, or grinding them into small pieces and place them in the cold water in your chosen cooking pot.

Allow the herbs to soak in the cold water for several hours.

Cover the pot and gradually bring it to a slow boil. Once boiling, reduce the heat to a gentle simmer.

Continue simmering until the liquid volume reduces to half of the initial amount, typically around 15-20 minutes. Strain the decoction using cheesecloth or a fine sieve. Once cooled, ensure to squeeze the herbs to extract all the liquid. Transfer the strained decoction into a jar with a secure lid for storage. Consume within 48 hours or freeze for longer preservation.

Decoctions boast a concentrated medicinal potency, containing approximately four times more active compounds than a standard herbal tea. For adults in good health, a dosage of up to 1 cup of decoction, taken three times a day, can be suitable, depending on the specific herb. Children's dosages should be adjusted based on their weight, typically reduced accordingly.

Double decoctions offer an even higher concentration of medicinal benefits. Similar to regular decoctions, they are simmered until the final volume equals ¼ of the original liquid volume, thus amplifying the medicinal concentration. Adults should limit their intake to 1 tablespoon of a double decoction, while children may consume up to ½ teaspoon for most herbs.

Double decoctions prove especially valuable when extracting compounds from shredded bark and dried roots, where the release of beneficial compounds occurs gradually. When working with these herbs, it's advisable to allow them to soak in cold water for 12 hours prior to boiling and simmering.

By employing these methods, one can harness the full therapeutic potential of herbs, tailoring dosages to individual needs and maximizing the efficacy of herbal remedies. ——————————————————

Oil Infusions

Infusing herbs into oil can be done through cold or hot methods. Cold extraction, which actually means room temperature, takes 6 to 8 weeks to fully infuse the herbs into the oil. The "hot" method, more accurately described as warm, involves gently heating the oil with herbs to expedite the process, suitable when a remedy is needed sooner. However, it's crucial to avoid boiling or overheating the oil to maintain the integrity of the herbal properties. Both methods offer benefits, and the choice depends on the herbs used and the desired timeframe for infusion.

Carrier Oils and "Cold" & "Hot" Infusions:

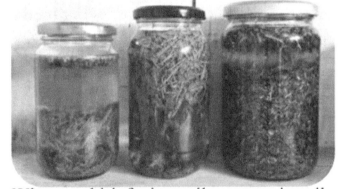

When cold-infusing oil, use primarily dried herbs to prevent spoilage from moisture. Opt for carrier oils like organic olive oil, preferred for its stability and suitability for salves. Ensure organic oils come from regions with strict labeling laws, such as California. Alternatives like sweet almond oil, coconut oil (note its temperature sensitivity), jojoba oil, and others work well too. Even rendered fats like bear fat can serve as bases for infusion.

1. Tear or crush dried herbs and lightly pack them into a clean, sterilized glass jar, filling it about 1/3rd full (for certain herbs like cottonwood buds or Usnea, fill it over half-full).

2. Pour high-quality organic olive oil or another natural plant oil over the herbs, filling the jar to within ½ inch (1.25 cm) of the top. Mix well to remove air bubbles, then cap and label the jar with the herb and date.

3. Place the jars in a crockpot and cook on low for 4 to 7 days, adjusting based on the herb. Ensure the water in the water bath/crockpot stays full. For fresh herbs, leave the caps off to allow moisture to evaporate, preventing water from entering the jars.

4. Once cooled, strain the herbs using cheesecloth or a tincture press, then pour the infused oil into a clean, sterile bottle or jar. This oil can be used directly for medicinal purposes or for making salves, and it typically lasts about 1 to 2 years.

Salve-making

Salves offer a practical method for applying herbs to the skin, effectively treating a variety of ailments such as burns, rashes, insect bites, wounds, eczema, muscle soreness, arthritis, and nerve pain. Converting herbal oil infusions into salves provides a convenient means of utilizing herbs on the go. To make a salve, you must first create an infused oil using the process outlined earlier. Alternatively, you can utilize the "fast method" below:

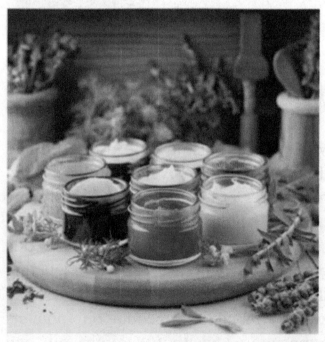

The fastest method for crafting herbal salves seamlessly integrates the infusion and salve-making stages.

It requires a generous amount of dried herbs. Begin by combining your herbs with enough oil to fully cover them in the top of a double boiler, ensuring there is water in the bottom half. Simmer gently for a few hours, maintaining a temperature of approximately 100 degrees Fahrenheit to avoid overheating. Stir the mixture, allow it to cool slightly, and strain it through cheesecloth. Return the infused oil to the double boiler and introduce melted beeswax, typically around 1/4 to 1/5 cup per cup of oil. Additionally, incorporate 15 to 20 drops or more of each essential oil per 8 ounces of oil for added therapeutic benefits. Consider adding vitamin E to prolong shelf life and prevent rancidity. Thoroughly mix the ingredients, pour the resulting blend into containers, and allow it to set.

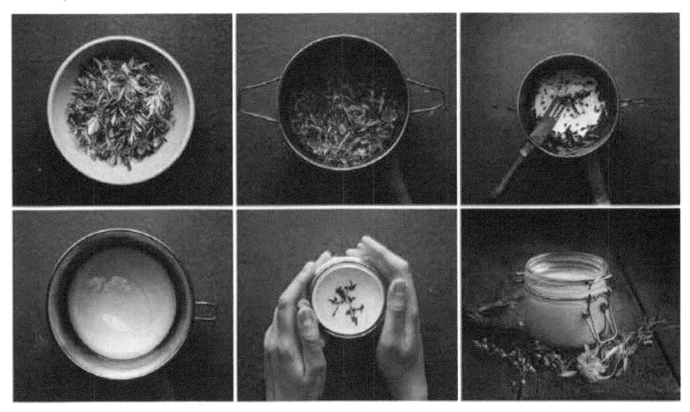

To craft a simple salve from your infused oil and beeswax:

1. Measure and pour your infused oil(s) into the top part of a double boiler.
2. Add beeswax and melt. I usually use a 1 part beeswax to 4 parts infused oil mixture and common usage is 1/4 cup to 1/5 cup per cup of oil. For 8 oz (250ml) of oil I use 2 oz (48g) of beeswax.
3. Mix together thoroughly until the beeswax has melted.

4. Add 15 to 20 drops or more of each of your essential oils for every 8 oz (250ml) of infused oil. Vitamin E can be added to help rancidity (1/2 tsp for 16 oz (250ml) oil). Add essential oils just before pouring.
5. Before you pour into your containers (jars/tins) to set you may add just a few drops to your container to test the consistency. If it's too hard add more oil and if it's too soft add more beeswax. Then complete pouring, label, and date

Tinctures/Extracts

Tinctures are medicinal extracts of any herb or herbal concoction in an alcohol, vinegar, or glycerin base. Because alcohol is a universal solvent, it is usually able to extract the essential oils from herbs, as well as extract most of the other chemical compounds that water is able to extract (note that some herbs need a double-extraction in water and alcohol to access all of the medicinal compounds).

But alcoholic tinctures have another, much more important attribute. They absorb into the body faster than any other means of using herbal medicines. This is due to the alcohol base, which starts absorbing through the stomach wall and even through the mouth upon taking the tincture. Rather than being digested, like other things that are eaten and drunk, the herbs are absorbed right into the bloodstream.

Another benefit of tinctures is that they last virtually forever, as long as they are stored in a well-sealed container. The alcohol is uniformly fatal to any microorganisms might that come into contact with it, so there is no possibility of the tincture decomposing. The biggest risk is evaporation.

To make a tincture you will need some sort of consumable alcohol that is at least 80 proof (40% alcohol). Vodka is the preferred alcohol to use, because it has no flavor, but rum, gin, brandy, and whiskey will work as well. You can also use apple cider vinegar or food grade vegetable glycerin, although these often don't work as well for many herbs and they don't last as long.

1. Fill a glass jar 1/3 to 1/2 full of the dried herbs you are using for your tincture, but don't pack it down (amount of the herb used depends on the surface area and extractability of the herb). You can also use fresh herbs – use 2x the amount of dried herbs.
2. Fill the jar with the alcohol, leaving ½ inch (1.25 cm) of headspace. Stir well.
3. Close the lid on the jar, label and date, and store in a cool, dry place. Tinctures can take anywhere from 4 weeks up to 6 months to fully extract, depending on the herbs you are using. 2 months works well for most herbs. Shake the jar once a day if possible.
4. Once your tincture is complete, usually around 8 weeks, strain out the herbs and rebottle the finished product. The alcohol renders it very shelf-stable and tinctures can last up to 7 years.

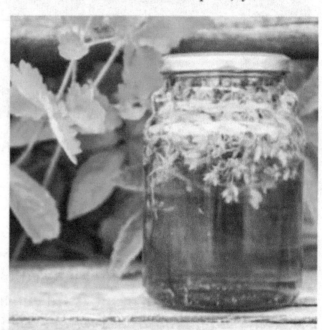

Double Extractions

A double extraction is a combination of a tincture and a decoction, often used for mushrooms and lichens. In recent years, the medicinal value of various types of mushrooms has been researched heavily. If only a water-based decoction is used with Reishi Mushroom, for example, it extracts the beneficial polysaccharides (including the beta-glucans) and the glycoproteins but not the triterpenes (like ganoderic acid in Reishi), as they are not soluble in water. Both water and alcohol are needed to extract all of the medicinal compounds.

For this tincture, alcohol and water are required. There are two methods. Both are below and different herbalists prefer different methods. Final alcohol percentage should be 25% to 30% or higher. The recipes below give you that percentage but you may also start with a higher proof alcohol. If you see cloudiness in your final product that is OK - it is just the polysaccharides coming out of solution. Simply shake before use.

Method #1: Starting with the alcohol extraction

Feel free to scale down this recipe. You'll need: 8 ounces (224g) or more of dried mushroom or lichen, 24 ounces (750ml) of 80 to 100 proof alcohol (40 to 50 % alcohol), 16 ounces (500ml) distilled water.

1. Fill a quart-sized (1 liter) canning jar half-full with diced dried mushrooms, then fill it to about ½ inch (1.25 cm) of the top with alcohol. Stir and cap it, shaking it every day for 2 months. Then strain out the alcohol and set it aside.
2. Make the decoction. Put 16 ounces (500ml) of water into a ceramic or glass pot with a lid and put the mushrooms into it. Cover and simmer the mixture until half of the water has boiled off. This will take a few hours. If the water level drops too quickly, add more so that you can continue simmering your mushrooms. The end result should be 8 ounces (250ml) of your decoction.
3. Allow the water to cool, and then strain out the mushrooms. Mix the water and alcohol (you should have about 24 oz (710ml) of alcohol tincture) together to create the finished double-extraction. It has a high enough alcohol content (30%) that it should be shelf-stable for many years, as long as it is stored in a sealed container.

Method #2 Starting with the water extraction

I like to use a small crockpot for this recipe. You may also place the herbs and water into a jar, which is then covered and placed into a crockpot of water on low or a pot of water on low on the stove. Feel free to scale down this recipe. You'll need: 8 ounces (230g) or more of dried mushroom or lichen, 24 ounces(710ml) of 80 to 100 proof alcohol, 16 ounces (500ml) distilled water.

1. Cut up the herbs into very small pieces. Place the distilled water and the dried herbs into the crockpot and stir well. Cover and cook on the lowest possible setting for 3 days. It will cook down to about 8 oz (250ml) of medicinal decoction (water).
2. Allow the herb and water mixture to cool and pour it into a large glass jar. Add the alcohol while the mixture is still quite warm, but not hot. Make sure the jar is large enough that you are adding 24 ounces (710ml) of alcohol or split everything evenly between 2 jars.
3. Cap the jar tightly, label and date the jar and allow it to macerate for 6 to 8 weeks, shaking the jar daily.
4. Strain out the herb (cheesecloth works well for this) or carefully decant the tincture off. Store it in tightly capped glass jar. Label and date.

Distillation

Distillation is a process used for extracting essential oils from herbs or other plants. Not all plants provide essential oils; but for those that do, this is one of the surer methods of extracting the essential oil.

Distillation is something that should only be undertaken by someone who wants to make a lot of essential oils, due to the equipment investment and the amount of plant matter you need. The amount of essential oil that is distilled out of plants is very small and it takes a pretty good size still to get enough oil to make the effort worthwhile. You may want to simply purchase organic essential oils from a reputable source to have on hand.

There are three basic types of distillation, requiring minor differences in the still:

❖ **Water distillation** – The herbs are immersed in water and the water is boiled. This works best for herbs that don't break down easily.

- **Water and steam distillation** – The only difference in the equipment for this and water distillation is the insertion of a rack inside the still, which holds the herbs up out of the water and only allows the steam to have contact with it. This method produces essential oils much more quickly than water distillation.

- **Direct Steam Distillation** – A different sort of still is needed for this method, so that the steam can be created in a separate chamber. The steam is then injected into the retort/still that is holding the herbs, below a rack holding the herbs. This allows a lower temperature to be used, reducing the potential for heat damage to the essential oil. This is the most common method used commercially, especially for essential oils like rosemary and lavender.

Much expertise is needed for distillation as the amount of plant material, distillation times, and temperatures are specific to the still and the herb from which you are trying to extract the essential oil.

Medicinal Syrups

Herbal syrups are a great way of getting children to take herbal medicines and supplements. Made with raw honey, they store extremely well, taste good, and can also soothe a sore throat. Making a medicinal honey syrup for treating colds, sore throats, or the flu will have the added benefit that the raw honey brings.

Before starting, decide how sweet you want your syrup. Some people like a sweeter syrup, using a 1:1 ratio of honey to decoction, while others use a 1:2 ratio, using less honey. The 1:1 ratio will store longer, as honey doesn't spoil easily. You can add glycerin in place of some of the honey to extend shelf-life.

To make any medicinal syrup, start out by making a decoction. You want to end up with a known amount of decoction, so that you'll know how much honey to add. This is easy, as you will need to strain out the herbs before adding the honey. When you do this, measure using a Pyrex glass measuring cup.

Typically, these syrups will last about six months in the refrigerator if you use a 1:2 ratio. You can also extend the life by adding a tincture to the mixture, as the alcohol in the tincture will act as a preservative, or by adding glycerin.

Poultices

Poultices may be one of the oldest ways in which herbal medicines are used. They provide an excellent way of applying healing herbs directly to the afflicted area. Usually used for first-aid field situations, such as dealing with burns, bee stings, cuts, and infections, they are also useful for deeper problems, like joint problems and bruises. They can even be applied to the chest to aid with congestion.

Normally, poultices are made of fresh herbs, picked on the spot. This means that they are at their most potent, able to provide the maximum possible benefit. They are also able to help draw out splinters, bee stingers, and other infection-causing foreign matter that has embedded itself into the skin.

One of the great things about poultices is that they are made on the spot to deal with a specific need. There is little preparation and they are not stored. Rather, they are often made of whatever herbs are readily available at the time. Of course, that requires the ability to recognize those herbs growing in the wild so that they can be harvested and put to use immediately.

How to Make a Poultice: To make a poultice, select the necessary fresh herbs and tear or cut them finely. If you don't have the ability to cut them, crushing them between the fingers will work too. Doctors carried a mortar and pestle in ancient times for this

purpose. The idea is to have the leaves broken, so that the sap of the plant can come out, contacting the skin. Chewing also works but make sure the herbs are safe to chew.

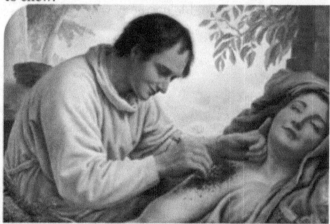

A generous quantity of the poultice is applied to the afflicted area of the skin and bound in place with a bandage. Gauze is normally used for this, but an elastic bandage or a large leaf are other options. The poultice must be kept damp to work, so it is usually changed out a couple of times per day.

Poultices can be made from dried herbs as well. In that case, the crushed or chopped herbs are soaked in warm water, softening them so that they won't irritate the skin and to draw out their medicine.

A little fine-tuning can be applied by using either hot or cold water with it. A hot poultice (not hot enough to burn) helps to increase the circulation in the area where it is applied. This can help get the medicinal properties of the herbs to the cells needing it more quickly. Using cold water, on the other hand, reduces circulation, while also reducing swelling.

How to Make a Field Poultice

Poultices have been used as field bandages and dressings for countless generations. In wartime, poultices helped manage many serious traumatic wounds and prevented as well as treated infection.

I have used poultices on both others and myself many times in the field. My most common go-to poultice herbs are Plantain, Yarrow, Mullein, and *Usnea*. I always carry dried Yarrow and Plantain with me in the winter when these plants are not readily available. These herbs are all in this book, so rest assured you'll have no problem identifying them. You can use these as single-herb poultices or mix them together.

One of my favorites is a plant growing in many back yards and probably yours as well: Plantain (*Plantago* spp.).

Plantain has a powerful antibacterial effect. It also contains allantoin, which is a phytochemical (a chemical found in plants) that speeds up wound healing and stimulates the growth of new skin cells. Plantain stops bleeding and helps relieve pain and itching. We use it for immediate relief for bites and stings.

Another common poultice herb is the plant known as "The Cowboy's Toilet Paper": Mullein. Mullein works in two different ways to enhance the effects of the plantain already in the poultice.

Mullein is an analgesic and thus lessens the pain, and it works as an astringent as well. That means it will

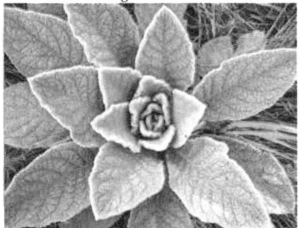

contract your skin and, in doing so, will help close the wound. This plant has the added benefit of being used as, well, toilet paper if you ever run out. It's very soft.

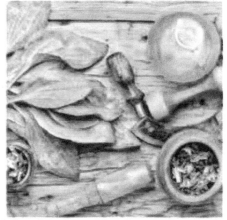

Another plant you can use alone or mix into your field poultice is Yarrow. Yarrow is a very strong anti-bacterial and is also a blood coagulant and thus helps stop bleeding.

Usnea Lichen is my other fantastic go-to for applying to a wound. It is very absorbent and has anti-microbial, anti-bacterial, anti-viral and anti-fungal properties. It is ready to go as is!

A strong herbal field poultice:

1. Gather plantain, mullein, and yarrow in equal quantities.
2. Grind the leaves together until you get a paste-like mixture. Add clean water if needed.
3. Apply it to your wound or cut.
4. Leave it on for one to two hours; then reapply as needed.
5. Keep the paste in place by using a non-toxic plant that has big leaves and high flexibility or normal bandages if you have some around. Burdock leaves are perfect for this if you don't have normal bandages.

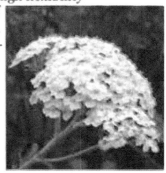

How to Make a Field Poultice

I do a lot to manage Multiple Sclerosis. This page is also available (with products links for your convenience) at www.nicoleapelian.com. I believe that a lot of this information can be extrapolated for other autoimmune conditions as well.

The first thing I did was get an IGG food sensitivity test to see how I needed to alter my diet for optimum health. I don't eat gluten. I also stick to a low sugar diet with few processed foods. I alternate an anti-inflammatory diet with a ketogenic diet and practice intermittent fasting. This works well for me. For some, a modified paleo diet is ideal. I find that adding freshly ground flax seeds into my diet is helpful. I have progressive Multiple Sclerosis (though it is not currently progressing!). Diet is really important in managing MS and health in general.

Here are some of the things I incorporate into my MS management in addition to diet:

I give gratitude daily and I try to stay in the present moment the best I can. (This is very important! The mind-body connection is huge.)

I spend time in nature daily. Nature connection is a big piece of total health for me.

I spend time away from media and carry a personal anti-EMF device and have another one for my home.

I take these specific vitamins and herbal remedies:

- ❖ High-dose Biotin & Alpha-Lipoic Acid. Personally, I take 100mg Biotin three times every day (300mg a day total) for progressive MS.
- ❖ 4000 units Vitamin D drops
- ❖ Omega 3s (and incorporate these into my diet)
- ❖ Multi--Vitamin + Ca/Mg blend
- ❖ Tru Niagen (nicotinamide riboside)
- ❖ Probiotics
- ❖ Vitamin B12 if my levels get low

For preventing general illness (which causes the dreaded immune response that then causes MS to flare up) I rely on my healing trinity of Elderberry Tincture, Usnea Spray, and First Aid Salve. You can make all of them using the information in this book.

The 3 tinctures that I take daily for MS are:

- ❖ Lion's Mane Mushroom Tincture. Lion's Mane is known to boost mental functioning and stimulate Nerve Growth Factor (NGF). Studies show great potential for myelination and regeneration of nerves.

- ❖ Reishi Mushroom Tincture. I make this tincture as a double-extraction. I take this daily as Reishi mushrooms are adaptogens, which help us deal with the negative effects of stress, address issues such as increased inflammation, depleted energy levels, damaged blood vessels, and various types of hormonal imbalances. Reishi has been shown to have neuroprotective effects and, because many autoimmune illnesses are inflammatory in nature, I also take it for its anti-inflammatory properties.

- ❖ Turkey Tail Mushroom Dual-extracted Tincture. I always make all of my products with locally sourced and/or organic ingredients. It works well for leaky gut, as turkey tail has prebiotics that helps balance the digestive system and helps with *Candida* overgrowth. It is also been shown to be a great cancer preventative, an anti-inflammatory, and more.

I keep leaky gut at bay. Plantain tincture works well for me for this as does Turkey Tail and probiotics. I do make a Leaky Gut Tincture, which can be found in my apothecary, and drink organic bone broth for my gut.

I keep internal inflammation down with my Reishi Mushroom Tincture and Turmeric.

Wishing you the best on your journey to health.

For more information and links to everything I discuss above please see www.nicoleapelian.com

Backyard Plants

Agrimony, *Agrimonia eupatoria*

Agrimony, also called sticklewort, cocklebur, or church steeples, is native to Europe and is now found across North America. It is a pretty plant with spikes of tiny yellow flowers. It is in the Rosaceae (Rose) Family.

Identification: This dark green perennial has a rough stem. It is covered with soft hairs that help it spread its seeds. It grows to a height of 2 feet (0.6meters).

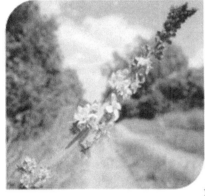

The leaves are serrated and pinnate. They are large (7 inches) (17.5 cm) at the base and get smaller at the top of the stem. Its roots are deep woody rhizomes.

The short-stemmed flowers have a sweet, apricot-like scent. They bloom from June to September on long terminal spikes. Each flower is a cup with rows of hook-shaped bristles on the upper edge. Flowers have five sepals and five yellow, rounded petals, each with 5 to 20 stamens.

The fruit has hooked bristles called cockleburs that attach to animals, thus spreading the seeds.

Edible Use: The leaves are used for tea, and the fresh flowers are often added to home-brewed beer or wine to enhance flavor.

Medicinal Use: Both the leaves and seeds are used in medicinal preparations. It is astringent, anti-inflammatory, and antibacterial.

To Induce Sleep: While lying in bed, place a few of this plant's leaves under your head to induce sleep.

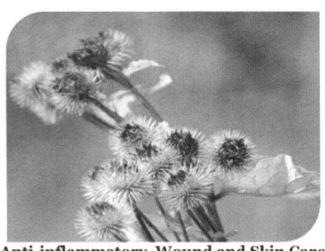

Anti-inflammatory, Wound and Skin Care: Agrimony is effective for wound care. It stops excessive bleeding by promoting the formation of clots. It contains tannins and is an astringent. It also has antibacterial and anti-inflammatory properties. Agrimony tea can be used as a wash for wounds and all types of skin diseases or the fresh leaves can be pounded and applied directly to a wound as a poultice.

Digestive Problems and Diarrhea: Agrimony Tea is used for digestive problems. The tea acts as a tonic to the digestive system and heals underlying problems.

Migraines: An herbal poultice made from fresh agrimony leaves and applied to the head is a good topical treatment for migraines. Use it at night as it may also induce deep sleep.

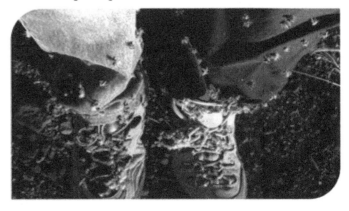

Conjunctivitis and Eye Infections: For application as an eye wash, mix equal parts of Agrimony Tea with boiled and cooled water.

Harvesting: Harvest agrimony in the late spring to early summer when the herb is in full bloom. Pick the leaves, flowers, and stems. Use the herbs fresh or dry them for later use.

Warning: Some people develop an allergic rash with sun exposure while using agrimony. Do not use if taking anti-coagulant therapy or taking blood-pressure medications. Avoid using agrimony if pregnant or nursing.

Recipes: Agrimony Tea. 1 to 2 teaspoons of powdered agrimony leaves or 3 teaspoons of crushed fresh leaves, 1 cup boiling water, raw honey, to taste, if desired. Steep the agrimony leaves in boiling water for 5 to 10 minutes. Cool and strain. Take one cup, three times daily.

Aloe Vera

Aloe Vera is edible and is incredibly effective for many afflictions. It's not native to North America, but it's been naturalized in many places. I find it readily in the southwest where the weather is warm and it is easy to grow in pots around the house. It is in the *Asphodelaceae* (Aloe) Family.

Identification: Aloe Vera plants have succulent leaves that grow to 2 to 3 feet (0.6 meters to 0.9 meters) tall.   The plant is stemless or has very short stems.   Aloe Vera leaves are thick, fleshy, and filled with gelatinous sap. The leaves grow in clumps, and are green to grey-green and may have white flecks on the leaf surfaces. The leaf margins are serrated with small white teeth. Flowers appear in the summer on a tall spike growing from the center of the plant. Flowers range in color from white and yellow to orange and red.

Edible Use: Eat aloe vera leaves raw or cooked. The outer green skin can also be eaten, but is bitter and tough. Removing the skin with a sharp knife leaves the meat and gel inside the plant; both are edible.

Aloe is good poached or otherwise gently cooked. Fully cooked, it loses its slimy texture. Some people enjoy raw aloe as juice or by putting a chunk in their water.

Medicinal Use: Aloe Vera gel, the gelatinous substance inside the leaf, is used as a relief for sunburn, wounds, and other minor skin irritations. It also has internal uses.

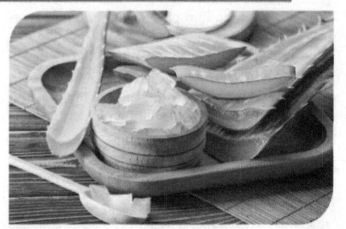

How to Use Aloe Vera: For external use, split the leaf long ways with a knife and scrape the gel from the leaf's interior. I most often use it as a soothing salve directly on the skin. For internal use, try 1 to 3 ounces (28-85g) of the gel added to juice, since the gel can be unpleasant and bitter when taken alone.

Heartburn Relief and Irritable Bowel Syndrome: Consuming 1 to 3 ounces (28g to 85g) of aloe vera gel with each meal reduces the severity of acid reflux and the associated heartburn. It also helps the cramping, abdominal pain, flatulence, and bloating caused by irritable bowel syndrome. However, there are some safety concerns and it may cause irritation, so use internally with care for these conditions.

Bleeding or Swollen Gums: Aloe Vera extract makes a safe and effective mouthwash that reduces swelling, soothes, and provides relief from bleeding or swollen gums. Try adding the gel to the final rinse water and swishing it around, holding it in the mouth for a minute, then spitting it out.

Lowering Blood Sugar in Diabetics: If you suffer from type 2 diabetes, you can regulate your blood sugar levels by simply ingesting two tablespoons of Aloe Vera juice or pulp extract daily.

Laxative: Aloe Vera gel relieves constipation but should be used sparingly.

Skin Care, Sunburn, Eczema: Aloe gel is soothing on the skin and an excellent remedy for sunburn, skin abrasions, eczema, and other mild skin irritations.

It also keeps skin clear and hydrated. Excellent as a moisturizer and pain reliever.

Warning: Long term internal use of Aloe Vera is not recommended due to the latex found in Aloe Vera. Do not use internally while pregnant. Do not use if you have hemorrhoids or kidney issues.

Anise Hyssop, *Agastache foeniculum*

Anise Hyssop is also known as blue giant hyssop, lavender giant hyssop, elk mint, and licorice mint. It belongs to the Lamiaceae (Mint) Family. It is native to northern and central North America.

Identification:

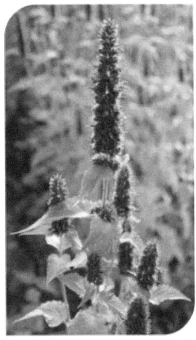

Anise hyssop grows from 2 to 5 feet (0.6 to 1.5m) tall, with bright green leaves that are notched at the edge and covered with fine white hairs on the underside. New growth has a purple tint. The plant has an aroma suggestive of mint and anise. The herb is partially woody with branched and usually hairless stems. The fibrous roots are also branching. Clusters of small lilac-blue flowers appear on elongated flower spikes from July through September.

Edible Use: Anise hyssop can be used as a sweetener and to make tea. It can be used as a flavoring or seasoning. The leaves and flowers can be eaten fresh, cooked, or dried.

Medicinal Use. Heart Healthy, Angina Pain: An infusion of anise hyssop is a tonic for the heart and a quick remedy for angina pain.

Sores, Wounds, and Burns: For skin infections, wounds, and burned skin, use a poultice of anise hyssop leaves. Soak dried leaves or bruise fresh leaves and flowers and apply them directly on the affected area. Cover with a clean cloth. Anise hyssop leaves have anti-bacterial and anti-viral properties.

Facilitates Digestion: Drinking Anise Hyssop Tea with meals eases digestion and prevents excessive gas and bloating.

Diarrhea: Anise hyssop tea is helpful in relieving diarrhea. The tea works best if continued throughout the day even after the diarrhea has been successfully eliminated. Continuing to sip occasionally prevents the return of diarrhea.

Sore Muscles and Anxiety: Try gathering 3 to 4 tablespoons of anise hyssop leaves in a square of cheesecloth and hang it from the faucet while drawing a bath. The scent released as the water flows calms the spirit. When the bath is ready, drop the herbs into the bathwater and soak your sore muscles in the bath.

Colds, Flu, Bronchial Congestion: Anise hyssop tea helps expel mucus from the lungs, making it a good choice for treating colds, flu, and congestion.

Herpes: Try Anise Hyssop Essential Oil externally as an antiviral treatment for Herpes Simplex I and II and drink the tea to treat the virus internally.

Poison Ivy: Wash the skin in Anise Hyssop Infusion to help relieve the itchiness of poison ivy.

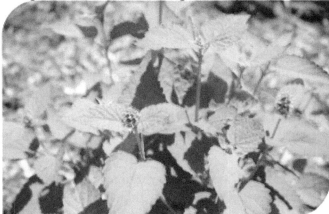

Athlete's Foot, Fungal Skin Infections, Yeast Overgrowth: Soak the foot or infected area in a bath with a strong infusion of Anise Hyssop. Soak daily until the infection is cured.

Recipes: Anise Hyssop Tea or Infusion. You'll need one cup of boiling water and raw honey to your liking. Add one teaspoon of dried leaves and flowers or one tablespoon of fresh leaves and flowers.

Add them to the boiling water and cover tightly. Allow the leaves to steep for 15 minutes.

Strain the tea through a fine sieve. Add raw honey to sweeten, if desired.

Ashwagandha, *Withania somnifera*

Ashwagandha, *Withania somnifera*, is a member of the nightshade family. It is sometimes called Winter Cherry or Indian Ginseng, due to its importance in Ayurvedic medicine. Ashwagandha is considered a rejuvenating adaptogenic herb, useful for treating many debilitating conditions.

Identification: Ashwagandha is native to India but can be grown in herb gardens across the United States. It is a perennial in warm climates with no frost. Ashwagandha likes sandy or rocky soil, full or partial sunlight, and moderately dry conditions.

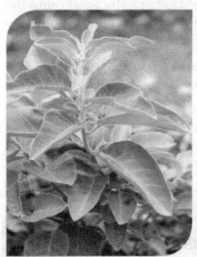

The bush grows to a height of 2 to 3 or more feet (0.6m-0.9m), with dull green leaves. Light green, bell-shaped flowers appear in midsummer and orange to red berries in the fall. Branches grow radially from a center stem.

Photo By Hari Prasad Nadig, CC BY 2.0

Edible Use: The plant is not generally eaten, but its seeds are used in the production of vegetarian cheeses. The leaves are used to make Ashwagandha Tea.

Other Uses: The fruits are rich in saponins are can be used as a substitute for soap. The leaves repel insects.

Medicinal Uses: Ashwagandha is an adaptogenic herb that has been in use for thousands of years. It is highly valued for its ability to strengthen the immune system, balance hormone levels, and for its anti-anxiety, anti-depressant, and anti-inflammatory properties. Roots and leaves of the ashwagandha plant are used for their medicinal properties.

Root extracts in powdered or capsule forms are effective as are leaf extracts and tinctures. Powders can be added to food or drinks thought they have a strong taste. Ashwagandha tea made from the leaves is also used. Adding a little honey improves the flavor.

Expect it to take two weeks or more to begin to notice the benefits of ashwagandha. Long-term use has not been studied and may not be safe, but many patients do well taking the herb long-term.

"Adrenal Fatigue" (= HPA Axis Dysregulation – HPA-D): Ashwagandha supports adrenal function and overcoming "adrenal fatigue", though this term is really a summary of stress response symptoms that are often caused by a hypothalamic–pituitary–adrenal (HPA) axis dysfunction. Essentially, HPA-D is our stress response system and a more accurate term for adrenal fatigue. Ashwagandha helps balance this.

Combats Stress, Fight or Flight, Anxiety, and Depression: Ashwagandha has long been used to relieve anxiety, improve mental health, concentration, vitality, and overall improve the quality of life. It also acts as a mood stabilizer and relieves symptoms of depression. It provides benefits similar to anti-anxiety and anti-depressant drugs without drowsiness, insomnia, or other side effects.

Reduces Cortisol Levels: Cortisol is a stress hormone implicated in controlling blood sugar levels and fat storage in the abdomen. Studies show that ashwagandha helps significantly reduce cortisol levels in chronically stressed adults.

Balances Blood Glucose Levels: Ashwagandha is particularly beneficial to diabetic patients in reducing blood glucose levels. It may help improve insulin sensitivity and reduce inflammation.

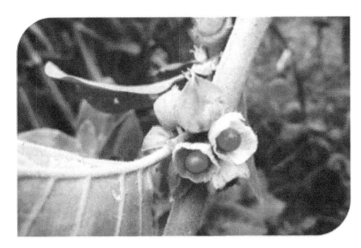

Cancer: Research shows that ashwagandha has anti-tumor effects. It reduces cancerous tumors by preventing cell growth and killing cancerous cells. Ashwagandha is useful in treating breast, lung, stomach, ovarian, and colon cancer cells. These benefits are due to its antioxidant abilities and their effects in helping the immune system.

In addition to reducing the growth of cancer cells, it can also help the body deal with the side effects of conventional anti-cancer drugs in boosting immunity and improving the quality of life. Ashwagandha stimulates the production of white blood cells and helps cancer patients fight infections.

Memory and Brain Cell Degeneration: Research suggests that ashwagandha protects the brain from the damaging effects of emotional, physical, and chemical stress. It protects the brain from cell degeneration, which may help in treating neurodegenerative diseases like Alzheimer's and Parkinson's Disease.

Ashwagandha contains naturally occurring steroids and antioxidants that protect the brain and improve cognitive function. Patients notice an improvement in attention, processing speed, and mental acuity.

Stamina, Endurance, and Muscle Performance: Studies suggest that ashwagandha boosts endurance and reduces muscle pain. It calms stress, energizes the brain, and enhances cardiorespiratory endurance in athletes. It increases muscle mass and strength in athletes engaging in resistance training and strenuous exercise when taken for 8-weeks or longer.

Anti-inflammatory: Joint Pain and Arthritis: Patients taking ashwagandha for eight weeks or longer experience improvement in joint function and a reduction in joint pain related to rheumatoid arthritis.

Sexual Function and Fertility: Ashwagandha helps improve sexual function. It boosts testosterone levels and improves male fertility. When used for a period of 3 months, ashwagandha increases sperm count, sperm volume, and sperm motility. In women, it improves arousal, lubrication, and orgasm.

Immune Function: Ashwagandha helps regulate immune function by reducing the body's stress hormones, reducing inflammation, increasing the white blood cell count, and increasing immunoglobulin production.

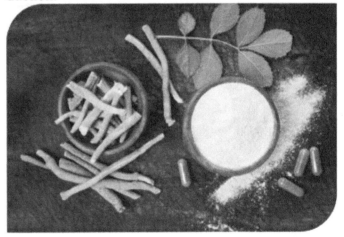

Harvesting: Pick berries in the fall when red and fully ripe, then dry them for planting in the spring. For medicinal use, dig up the roots in the fall and clean thoroughly. Slice, dry, and powder for future use. Leaves are used fresh or can be dried to use in tea.

Warning: The herb is generally believed to be safe and has an extensive history of use. However, there are no long-term studies on the safety and long-term use may make it more likely that side effects will be experienced. Consult your doctor and watch for side-effects when using ashwagandha over the long term.

Black-Eyed Susan, *Rudbeckia hirta*

Black-eyed Susan is a member of the Aster/Sunflower Family, and is found throughout eastern and central North America. It is also called brown-eyed Susan, hairy coneflower, gloriosa daisy brown betty, yellow daisy, yellow ox-eye daisy coneflower, poor-land daisy, and golden Jerusalem. It prefers full sun and moist to moderately-dry soil.

Identification: Black-eyed Susan is usually an annual; but sometimes a perennial, growing up to 3 feet (0.9m) tall and up to 1 ½ feet (0.5m) wide.

The leaves are alternate, 4 to 7 inches (10 cm to 20 cm) long, and covered by coarse hair. The branched stems grow from a single taproot.

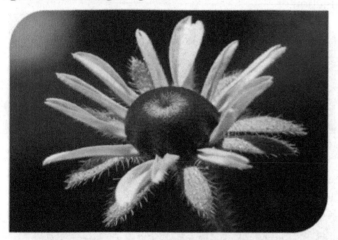

There is no rhizome and reproduction is by seed only. Be on the lookout for these flowers during late summer and early autumn. They are about 4 inches (10 cm) in diameter, with a brownish black dome in the middle, circled by yellow petals.

Medicinal Use: Black-eyed Susan is a traditional herb used for colds, flu, infection, swelling, and snake bite. The roots and sometimes the leaves are used to boost immunity and fight colds, flu, and infections.

Colds and Flu: A root infusion treats colds and the flu. Common usage is to drink the root infusion daily until all symptoms are gone.

Parasites: The Chippewa people have traditionally used Black-eyed Susan Root Tea to treat worms in children.

Poultice for Snake Bites: A poultice of black-eyed Susan is said to treat snakebites. Moisten the hopped leaves or ground root and place over the affected area as a poultice. Wrap with a cloth and keep it on the wound until the swelling is reduced.

Skin Irritations: Black-eyed Susan root infusions are soothing on irritated skin including sores, cuts, scrapes, and swelling. Use a warm root infusion to wash the irritated skin.

Earaches: If you have fresh roots, use the sap or juice as drops to treat earaches. One or two drops in the affected ear treat the infection and relieves pain. Place the drops in the ear morning and night until the infection is completely cleared up.

Stimulates the Immune System: Like Echinacea, Black-eyed Susan roots have immune-stimulant activity and boost the immune system to treat colds, flu, and other minor illness. Those with autoimmune issues should be careful using this herb internally due to its immune-stimulating properties.

Tuberculosis: Black-eyed Susan contains compounds that act against the bacterium that causes tuberculosis.

Harvesting: To harvest the taproot, wait until the plant has produced seeds, then dig the plant up by the root. Black-eyed Susan has one central taproot with hairs, but no other rhizomes. Dig deeply to get the entire root. Use it fresh in season and also dry some root for future use.

Warning: Black-eyed Susan plants are toxic to cats and are reported to be poisonous to cattle, sheep, and pigs. The seeds are poisonous. Those with autoimmune conditions should be careful with internal use of this herb due to its immune-stimulating properties.

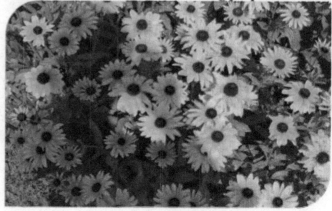

Boneset,
Eupatorium perfoliatum

This herb supposedly got the name boneset due to its use treating dengue fever, also known as break-bone fever. It is excellent for treating fevers and is a great choice for chest colds and flu. The herb is a perennial native to North America. It is a member of the Aster/Sunflower family. It is also known as feverwort.

Identification: Boneset has erect, hairy stems that grow 2 to 4 feet (0.6m to 1.2m) high and branch at the top. The leaves are large, opposite, and united at the base. They are lance-shaped, finely toothed and have prominent veins. Leaves are 4 to 8 inches (10 cm to 20 cm) long with the lower ones larger than the upper ones. The blades are rough on the top and downy, resinous, and dotted on the underside.

The leaves of boneset are easily distinguished. They are either perforated by the stem or connate; two opposite leaves joined at the base.

The numerous large flower heads of boneset are terminal and slightly convex, with 10 to 20 white florets, and have bristly hairs arranged in a single row.

The fragrance is slightly aromatic, while the taste is astringent and strongly bitter. Flowering from July to September, this plant's size, hairiness and other aspects can vary greatly.

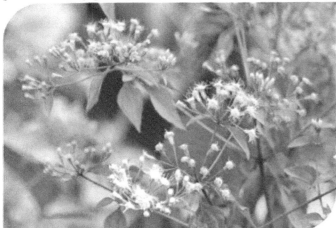

Medicinal Use: The flowers and leaves are used. Best to let dry rather than use fresh due to some degree of toxicity. The major medicinal properties of boneset include use as an antispasmodic, sweat inducer, bile-producer, emetic, fever-reducer, laxative, purgative, stimulant, and as a vasodilator.

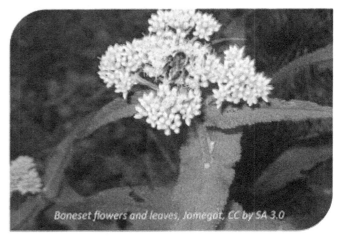
Boneset flowers and leaves, Jomegat, CC by SA 3.0

Colds, Flu, Bronchitis, Congestion and Excess Mucus: Boneset is an excellent choice for the treatment of the common cold, flu, and respiratory infections. It discourages the production of mucus, loosens phlegm and helps eliminate it from the body, fights off both viral and bacterial infections, and encourages sweating, which helps reduce the associated fever.

People given boneset early in the disease process have milder symptoms and get well faster. A tincture is the easiest form to use.

Dengue Fever, AKA Break Bone Fever: Dengue fever thrives in tropical environments, and while it is not yet a problem here in the United States, it is probably only a matter of time before it arrives.

Boneset is the herb of choice for fighting dengue, a painful mosquito-borne disease that results in high fevers and terrible muscle and bone pain. It reduces the fevers and fights the underlying causes of the disease. It also gives the patient some relief from the "bone-breaking" pain.

Malaria: Native Americans have commonly used boneset to treat malaria. It promotes sweating, which helps relieve the fever associated with malaria and lessens the severity of the disease.

Yellow Fever and Typhoid: Boneset is helpful in the treatment of yellow fever and typhoid, although it is not as effective as it is for treating dengue fever and malaria. Its main use here is its ability to reduce the accompanying fevers.

Harvesting: Harvest the leaves and flowering stems of boneset during the summer, just before the buds have opened. Dry them for later use. Seeds of boneset ripen about a month after flowering and are collected when the heads are dry, split, and the fluffy seed begins to float away. If seeds are collected earlier, dry the seed heads for 1 to 2 weeks in open paper bags.

Warning: Do not use boneset for pregnant or nursing mothers or for young children. Not for long-term use.

Recipes: Boneset Infusion. Take Boneset Infusion hot to relieve fevers and treat colds, flu, and similar diseases. Use it cold as a tonic or tincture.

Ingredients: 1-ounce dried boneset leaf, 1-quart (1 Liter) boiling water, 1-quart (1 Liter) jar with a tight-fitting lid.

Instructions: Put the dried boneset leaves into the jar and pour the boiling water over it to fill the jar. Tightly cap the jar and shake it gently to distribute the herb.

Let the infusion steep for 4 hours. Strain through a coffee filter or a fine sieve. Warm it before drinking. It is very bitter, but warming it helps.

Borage, *Borago officinalis*

Common Borage is an annual frequently found in gardens. Bees are attracted to the flowers and make an excellent honey from the nectar.

Identification: The entire borage plant is covered with stiff white hairs. The stems are round, branched, hollow, and succulent. The plant grows to about 1 1/2 feet tall. Its deep green leaves are alternate, wrinkled, oval and pointed. Each is about 3 inches long and about 1 1/2 inches across. The lower leaves have tiny hairs on the upper surface and on the veins on the lower side. Leaf margins are wavy, but entire.

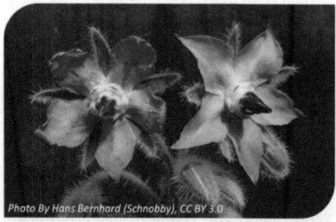
Photo By Hans Bernhard (Schnobby), CC BY 3.0

The flowers are a vivid blue and star-shaped, with prominent black anthers. The anthers form a cone in the center that is referred to as a beauty spot. The flowers start pink and turn blue, hanging in clusters.

The flowers produce four brown-black nutlets.

Edible Use: The leaves, flowers, dried stems, and seeds are all edible and nutritious. You can eat the leaves raw or cooked. I use them in salads or cooked as

a pot-herb. The leaves have a salty flavor similar to a cucumber. It is best to use the leaves while young. The more mature raw leaves are very hairy, which some people find unpleasant.

The flowers are nice used raw as a decorative garnish for salads and drinks. They make a refreshing drink when the leaves are brewed as a tea.

Dried stems are often used as a flavoring. The seeds are a healthy source of gamma-linolenic acid (GLA), a beneficial Omega-6 fatty acid, but it is difficult to collect enough for regular use.

Medicinal Use. Regulates Hormones, PMS and Menstrual Issues: Borage treats hormonal imbalances and regulates metabolism. Eating borage with meals regularly helps keep your metabolism running smoothly.

Borage reduces symptoms of premenstrual syndrome (PMS), menopause, and regulates the menstrual cycle.

Stress and HPA-Dysfunction ("Adrenal Fatigue"): Borage is a calming herb and is taken to relieve stress. It also helps balance cortisol levels in the body, this aiding the stress response and HPA-Dysfunction (often called Adrenal Fatigue).

Anti-Oxidant Properties: Anti-oxidants in borage helps destroy free radicals in the body, protecting it against aging and cancers caused by free radicals.

Digestive Problems and Irritable Bowel Syndrome: Borage has a soothing effect on the stomach muscles and is a good treatment for irritable bowel syndrome.

It reduces inflammation in the intestinal tract and treats gastritis and other digestive problems. It promotes digestion and stabilizes the stomach. Borage also has a mild laxative effect.

Pneumonia: Borage Leaf and Flower Tea or Tincture reduces the symptoms of pneumonia, relieves congestion, and helps the body get rid of excess mucus. However, there are better herbs for these symptoms.

Mouth Ulcers and Sore Throats: Use borage as a mouthwash or gargle to kill bacteria in the mouth and throat. It prevents and treats sore throats and mouth sores.

Urinary Tract and Kidney Infections, Diuretic Properties: Borage acts as a diuretic, removing excess water and toxins from the body. It also works to improve bladder function. Borage flushes the bladder, removing bacteria and relieving bladder infections. Borage also relieves kidney inflammations and restores health of the kidneys. However, I prefer other herbs to treat these, such as Usnea, Oregon Grape and Uva Ursi.

Protects the Brain: The GLA in borage seed oil improves the brains protection against neuro-degeneration. It protects the brain against synaptic failure in Alzheimer's disease and improves resistance to the disease.

Lowers Blood Pressure: Eat borage or drink the juice daily to treat high blood pressure. The GLA content helps to significantly lower blood pressure. Recent studies have confirmed the benefits of Borage for treating hypertension.

Allergies: The anti-oxidants in borage help subdue allergies, reduce inflammation, and suppress the allergic response.

Reduces Fevers: Borage stimulates the sweat glands to produce sweat and cool the body. This property is beneficial for treating fevers in colds, and respiratory illnesses.

Arthritis and Gout: Borage is useful for treating inflammation, reducing swelling, and thereby reducing pain. It is effective for reducing inflammation caused by arthritis and gout.

Skin Infections, Wounds, and Rashes: The anti-inflammatory and anti-bacterial properties of borage help keep your skin clear. It is useful in treating wounds and fighting infections or rashes. Use borage tea as a skin wash or use borage as a poultice to treat wounds. A poultice of borage leaves also reduces itching and inflammation from rashes or stings and insect

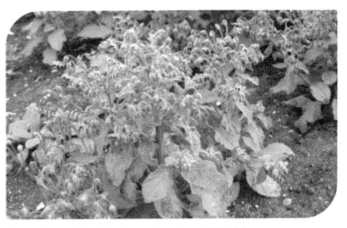

Photo By David Wright, Geograph project, CC BY 2.0

bites. It clears up skin inflammations and the unpleasant symptoms of skin rashes.

Treating Bleeding Gums: Borage fights the infections that cause bleeding gums. Borage helps kill the mouth pathogens and restores health to the gums and mouth.

Macular Degeneration: One cause of macular degeneration is a lack of fatty acids. Borage seeds contain up to 30% GLA, a beneficial fatty acid for treating and preventing macular degeneration.

Improves Milk Production for Nursing Mothers: Borage tea is used to improve milk production in nursing mothers.

Treat Hangovers: Borage Tea made from a combination of dried leaves and flowers is an effective treatment for hangover.

Harvesting: Harvest borage leaves in the late spring and early summer before the plant flowers. Use the leaves fresh or dry them for use throughout the year. Dried leaves lose their medicinal properties over time, so dry a new batch each year. Harvest flowers in the morning in the summer.

Warning: Borage leaves contain a small amount of pyrrolizidine alkaloids and other compounds that are toxic to the liver.

The levels are low and are not a problem for healthy people, but people with liver disease should not use borage in any form. Pregnant women should avoid using borage. In some people, borage causes skin dermatitis. Persons with schizophrenia or epilepsy should avoid using borage.

Bottle Gourd, *Lagenaria siceraria*

Also known as calabash, white-flowered gourd, and long melon, the bottle gourd is often cultivated for its fruit. When harvested young, the fruit is used as a vegetable. When mature, it is dried, and it can be scraped and used as a bottle, container, or pipe. Bottle gourd is in the cucumber family. It is hard to find in the wild, but easy to cultivate.

Identification: This annual vine grows to be 15 feet (4.5m) long or more. The fruit has a smooth light-green skin and white flesh. It grows in a variety of shapes and sizes. It has long densely packed hairs on the stems.

These hairs are tipped with glands that produce a sticky sap. The leaves grow on long stalks and are oval to heart-shaped. Leaves can be unlobed or have 3 to 5 irregular shallow lobes. The flowers are white, growing alone or in pairs. They open at night during the summer and close again in the morning.

Edible Use: Although it is safe to eat in moderate amounts, be aware that young gourds can be bitter. If you think the plant has grown too old or tastes too bitter, throw it away because it might have a buildup of toxins or it may have spoiled. Otherwise, the fruit can be steamed, boiled, fried, used in soups and stir-fries. Young shoots and leaves are cooked as a pot herb.

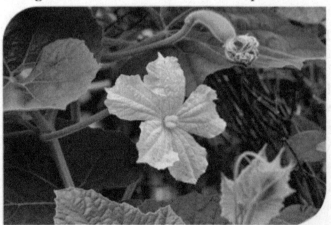

Medicinal Use: This plant is mainly used for blood sugar control in diabetics, but I know of healers who use it as a heart tonic and as a sedative. It is anti-inflammatory, antioxidant, anti-bacterial, pain relieving, and a tonic for the internal organs.

Diabetes: Bottle gourd helps to lower blood sugar readings in diabetics when taken regularly. Eat a piece of bottle gourd at each meal for blood sugar control. One or two large bites of the gourd are enough to provide the desired benefit.

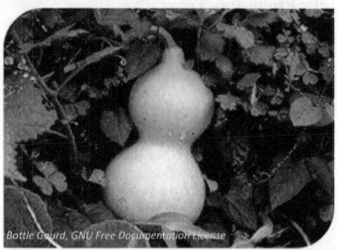

Bottle Gourd, GNU Free Documentation License

Headaches: A poultice made by crushing the leaves and applying it to the head over the painful area is useful for relieving the pain of headaches.

Boils, Skin Infections, and Irritations: Bottle gourd has anti-bacterial and anti-inflammatory effects. For these external uses, make poultice from the boiled seeds of the gourd for skin irritations and infections.

Cover the poultice with a clean cloth and leave in place as long as possible to reduce swelling and prevent the spread of the infection.

Memory Loss, Depression and Senility: Studies have been done demonstrating bottle gourd for mild depression and memory improvement, including patients with Alzheimer's Disease and age-related senility.

Cabbage, *Brassica oleracea*

The common cabbage is familiar to gardeners across the country, but many don't realize how valuable it is as a medicinal plant. The plant is a biennial or perennial, forming a round head that can reach up to 8 feet (2.4m) when fully mature. Most cabbages are harvested long before they reach such a size. It is in the Brassicaceae (Mustard) Family.

Identification: The leaves are gray with a thick stem. Yellow flowers with four petals appear in the spring. The leaves form a head during the late summer of the first year. Cabbage can also be reddish-purple, green, or white. All varieties have the health-giving benefits detailed below.

Edible Use: The cabbage is a common vegetable, especially in the winter because it keeps well in the root cellar. It is eaten raw and cooked.

Medicinal Use. Mastitis and Painful Breasts in Nursing Mothers:
This is my number one use for cabbage leaves. For painfully engorged breasts and mastitis, use a poultice made from cabbage leaves. Cut out the vein from the cabbage leaf and crush or pound the leaf with a hammer. You'll want your leaf intact but badly bruised to access the healing sulfur compounds and the juice. Apply the bruised leaf to the breast or line the bra cup with the leaf. Repeat as needed until the infection clears.

Treatment for Wounds, Leg Ulcers, Joint Pain, Arthritis, Skin Cancers:
Cabbage leaves work well to clean wounds and prevent infection. They are also useful in reducing swelling in painful joints and treating skin tumors.

Chop the leaves and crush them to release the health-giving juices and heat them in a very small amount of water. Apply the leaves as a poultice over the affected area. The cabbage detoxifies the skin and underlying tissue, prevents bacterial growth, and reduces inflammation.

Intestinal Problems: Cabbage is useful for treating intestinal problems due to its sulfurous compounds. Fermented cabbage in the form of sauerkraut is even more effective for treating intestinal problems of all kinds.

Diabetes: Sauerkraut juice, mixed with a little lemon juice, helps people control their diabetes and stabilize their blood sugars. The sauerkraut juice stimulates the digestion and pancreas.

Constipation: Cabbage, cabbage juice, and sauerkraut juice all have laxative properties.

Treating Cancer: For treating cancer, especially cancers of the stomach, intestines, pancreas, and prostate, drink cabbage juice or sauerkraut juice twice daily. Finely chopped cabbage should also be eaten as tolerated. Both cabbage juice and sauerkraut juice have many different beneficial compounds that fight cancer and help heal the body.

Recipes: Sauerkraut. Equipment: Large glass jar or crock. I prefer using a fermentation crock, but a glass jar will work, a fermentation weight or a plate that fits in the container, a large bowl or tub for mixing, a plate or tray. Ingredients for 1 gallon (4 liters) of Sauerkraut: 1 large head of cabbage, shredded fine, a few large leaves from the outside of the cabbage, 3 tablespoons pickling salt and 1 tablespoon caraway seeds, optional.

Shred the cabbage finely and add 2 TBS of salt. Let the cabbage stand for about 10 minutes to draw out juices. Knead the cabbage for 10 minutes or more to bruise it and release more juices.

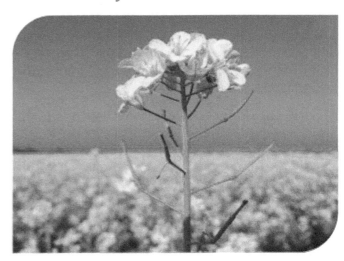

Cabbage, By Taken byfir0002, GFDL 1.2

Add the remaining salt and the caraway seeds. Pack the cabbage into a large glass jar or crock and add the juices. Cover the top of the shredded cabbage with the whole cabbage leaves. Add a weight to the top of the cabbage to keep it beneath the liquid.

Fermenting crocks use fermenting weights, but a clean plate or another dish can be used. Cover the container with its lid. Place the container in a cool spot on a tray or plate to catch any spills. Leave the cabbage overnight and check it the next day to make sure that all the cabbage is submerged in liquid and skim off any scum that forms.

Continue checking the sauerkraut every other day for 4 weeks. Transfer the sauerkraut to the refrigerator and use within 6 months. Sauerkraut can be canned for longer storage. However, I believe this destroys some of the beneficial enzymes as well as the live culture. I recommend using the sauerkraut with live culture.

Calendula, *Calendula officinalis*

Calendula or Pot Marigold is a perennial plant in the Aster/Daisy family that is often grown as an annual. It is not originally native to North America but is widely cultivated in flower gardens, self-seeds, and is easy to grow.

Identification: Calendula usually grows 12 to 24 inches (30 cm to 60 cm) tall with branched sprawling or erect stems. The leaves are oblong and lance-like, approximately 2 to 7 inches (5 cm to 18 cm) long, and hairy on both sides. The margins can be smooth, wavy, or even weakly toothed.

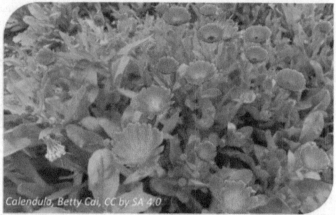
Calendula, Betty Cai, CC by SA 4.0

The flowers are yellow or orange with a 2 to 3-inch (5 cm to 7.5 cm) flower head with two rows of hairy bracts. Flowers appear year-round in warmer climates. Some flowers have multiple rows of ray florets while others have only one. High resin varieties and multi-row flowers are said to be better for medicine. The fruit is a small curved achene.

Edible Use: Calendula flowers are edible raw in salads or dried and used as a seasoning. They can be used as a saffron substitute for color but not taste. Tea is made from the petals. The leaves are edible, but are bitter and unpalatable.

Medicinal Use: Calendula can be used as a tea, infused oil, salve, compress, or poultice.

Skin Diseases, Cuts, Rashes, Wounds, Burns, Cold Sores, Herpes, Chicken Pox, and Irritations: Calendula leaves and flowers are soothing to the skin, and I use them to treat all kinds of skin problems like acne, sunburn, and rashes, including diaper rash. The leaves make a healing poultice for minor cuts, scratches, bites, and skin irritations.

Place the bruised leaves directly on the skin. The leaves soothe inflamed skin and help it heal. I use the flowers to make a healing salve for skin irritations. The leaves and flowers have anti-bacterial, anti-fungal, anti-microbial, and anti-viral effects as well being an immunostimulant. To treat skin infections, including ringworm, athlete's foot, thrush, diaper rash, and cradle cap, I use Calendula Oil or Salve applied to the affected area several times a day. Note that Calendula is a tonic anti-fungal, weaker than many. I prefer to use a stronger anti-fungal such as black walnut hull powder, Oregano Oil, or Usnea to treat the primary infection and save calendula as a preventative or for chronic situations.

Anti-aging and Collagen Production: Calendula stimulates the immune system, induces collagen production and inhibits collagen degradation. I make an anti-aging blend with Calendula and Cottonwood Buds infused in organic almond oil and use it on my face and neck every day in place of a commercial face cream.

Soothes Muscle Spasms: Calendula relaxes muscles and can prevent spasms. Calendula tea treats abdominal cramping caused by constipation and menstrual cramping.

It is also effective in relieving body aches and pains due to muscle spasms.

Helps Heal Ulcers, Wounds, and Hemorrhoids: Slow healing wounds such as ulcers and hemorrhoids are soothed by the application of calendula as an ointment, gel, or salve. It speeds up healing and wound closure while improving skin firmness and hydration. Calendula increases the blood and oxygen availability in the infected area, which encourages rapid healing. It is antimicrobial and antibacterial.

Stomach and Intestinal Diseases: Calendula works to heal a variety of gastro-intestinal problems including intestinal colitis, GERD, esophageal irritation, peptic ulcers, and inflammatory bowel disease. It soothes the inflammation from infections and irritations while helping heal the underlying problems.

Immune System and Lymphatic System: Calendula stimulates the functioning of the immune system and the lymphatic system, including swollen lymph nodes and tonsillitis, and helps to prevent infections.

Additionally, the astringent and antiseptic properties help the body fight off infections and viruses. Calendula also reduces congestion and swelling in the lymph glands.

Menstruation and PMS: Calendula Tea is an effective aid in easing the painful side effects of menstruation. It helps induce the menses, relieves painful cramping, relaxes the muscles, and improves blood flow. Some people claim that it also helps with hot flashes.

Improves Oral Health: Calendula has powerful antibacterial and antimicrobial properties and treats gingivitis, plaque, oral cavities and many other oral health issues.

Inhibits Cancer: Calendula has anti-inflammatory properties which aid the body in fighting cancer, as well as irritations caused by cancer treatments. It activates the lymphatic system against the cancer and helps kill off the cancer cells. It also effectively soothes the skin after radiation treatments.

Liver, Gallbladder, and Whole-Body Detoxification: Calendula helps remove toxins from the body and helps cleanse the liver and gallbladder. The detoxification properties also have a positive effect on the skin and help clear up chronic skin problems such as eczema and acne caused by the body's efforts to rid itself of toxins. For detoxification, try an internal Calendula Extract.

Harvesting: To promote flowering, pick the flowers every two days. Dry them on screens or hang them in a well-ventilated warm area.

Warning: Some people are allergic to calendula. Do not use it if you are allergic to marigold, ragweed, daisies, chrysanthemums, chamomile, echinacea and other plants in the Aster/Daisy family. If you are not sure, start with a small test patch on the skin and increase use gradually if you have no reactions. Do not use calendula internally if you are pregnant or breastfeeding, since safety is unknown. Do not take calendula internally if you are taking prescription medications without the advice of your doctor.

Recipes: Soothing Calendula Salve (Fast Method). Ingredients: half a cup of organic olive oil, 1/3 cup solid organic coconut oil, 3 tablespoons dried calendula flowers, 1 1/2 tablespoons dried chamomile flowers, 1 to 2 ounces (28g to 56g) beeswax. In a double boiler, melt the olive oil and the coconut oil together.

Add the flower petals and allow the mixture to steep for 2 to 3 hours making sure it does not get too hot. Strain out the flower petals. Return the pan to the heat and add the beeswax, stirring. Once the wax melts pour into your containers (adjust amount of beeswax to get the consistency you want). Allow the salve to cool completely before use.

Calendula Extract: Take 1-pint (500ml) loosely packed calendula flowers and 1-pint (500ml) 80 proof vodka or other drinking alcohol of 80 proof or higher. Place the flowers in a pint (500ml) jar with a tight fitting lid.

Fill the jar with alcohol so that the flowers are completely covered.

Allow the extract to steep in a cool, dark place for 4 to 6 weeks. Shake daily. Strain out the flowers and store the extract tightly covered in a cool, dark place. Use within 3 years.

California Poppy, *Eschscholzia californica*

The California poppy has sedative and healing effects but is not psychoactive or narcotic like some poppy species.

The California poppy is a species of flowering plant in the Papaveraceae (Poppy) Family, It is native to Western North America. It occurs across a variety of habitats including coastal, foothill, valley, and desert regions, at elevations below 7000 feet (2133m). It is also known as Golden Poppy and Cup of Gold due to its golden color.

Identification: The California poppy is a flowering annual or deep-rooted perennial. It is 1/2 to 2 feet (0.6m) tall, and its foliage is blue-green in color. Its leaves are compound, with three finely divided lobes, and are nearly smooth with no hair.

California poppy produces upright flowers on branching stems with four bright orange to yellow petals. The flowers often have distinct, darker orange centers.

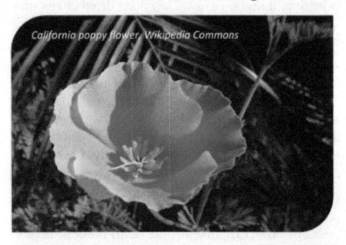
California poppy flower, Wikipedia Commons

The seed capsules of California poppy are cylindrically shaped and burst open from the base when ripe. These capsules open explosively to aid in seed dispersal, ejecting the small seeds up to 6 feet (1.83m) from the parent plant. Its tiny round seeds are usually gray to gray-brown in color when mature.

Edible Use: Its leaves are edible if cooked. Caution is advised because other plants in the family are poisonous.

Medicinal Use: The California poppy is a diuretic, relaxes spasms, relieves pain, promotes perspiration,

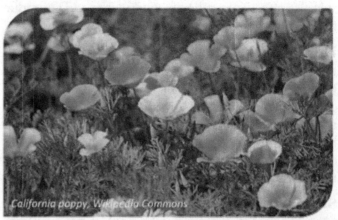
California poppy, Wikipedia Commons

and is sedative. It is non-addictive and can help with opiate withdrawal. It most likely works with GABA receptors. The entire plant is used medicinally, with the root being the most potent part.

Sedative Properties and Antispasmodic: California poppy is a mild sedative that also works well for incontinence, especially for children. It aids in treating sleep deprivation, anxiety, and nervous tension. The sap is somewhat narcotic and works well for alleviating toothaches. Unlike opium poppy, it does not depress the nervous system and it's much milder in action. Take it at bedtime since it induces sleep. It is also an antispasmodic.

Normalizes Psychological Function, PTSD, and Anxiety: California poppy seems to normalize the thinking patterns of people with psychological issues, and is mild enough to use for children. It does not have a narcotic effect, but helps calm the spirit and helps people regain normal function. It works well for anxiety disorders and PTSD.

Suppresses the Milk in Nursing Mothers: When lactation is not desired, apply California Poppy Tea made from the roots as a wash on the breasts to suppress the flow of milk. It helps the milk dry up quickly.

Harvesting: Harvest the entire plant when it is flowering from June to September and dry for use in tinctures and infusions.

Warning: Do not drive or operate heavy machinery, as it is a sedative.

Recipes. California Poppy Infusion: 1 to 2 teaspoons of dried California poppy plant or root, 1 cup boiling water. Make a strong tea by infusing the dried herb in boiling water for 10 minutes and allowing it to cool. Drink one cup of the infusion at night before going to bed. It induces sleepiness.

California Poppy Tincture: 1-pint (500 ml) of 80 proof vodka or other alcohol, or substitute apple-cider vinegar, dried or fresh California poppy plant.

Place the chopped fresh herbs or dried plant into a pint (500ml) jar with a tight-fitting lid, filling the jar 3/4 full. Cover the herbs with alcohol, filling the jar. Store the jar in a cool, dark place such as a cupboard. Shake the jar daily for 4 to 6 weeks. Strain the herbs out of the liquid, cover it tightly and use within seven years.

Carolina Geranium, *Geranium carolinianum*

Geranium carolinianum, known as Carolina Geranium, Carolina Cranesbill, Crane's Bill Geranium, and Wild Geranium, is native across the US, Canada, and Mexico.

This plant is often found in areas with poor soil, clay, and limestone. I often see it near roadsides, abandoned fields, and farmland.

Identification: The Carolina geranium is a winter annual or biennial herb. It is low-growing, usually under 12 inches tall. It has earned the name cranesbill because of the beak-like appearance of the fruit. Its palmate leaves have 5 to 7 toothed lobes, with each lobe divided again.

Leaves are 1 to 2.5 inches (2.5 cm to 6 cm) wide, grayish-green and covered in fine hair. Each leaf usually has five segments, edged with deep teeth. Its pinkish-red stems grow erect and are covered in hairs.

White, pink, or lavender flowers appear in small clusters on stalks growing off the main stems in April through July. Each flower has five sepals and five notched petals.

One-half inch long fruits, with a longer style, ripen in the fall. Ripe seeds are covered in pits/depressions.

The plant has a taproot system that grows close to the surface.

Edible Use: Carolina Geranium is edible raw, cooked, or as a tea. The roots are best boiled for 10 minutes to soften. The cooking water can be used as a tea to relieve stomach upsets.

The leaves are astringent and have a strong bitter flavor caused by their high tannin level. Using them young helps relieve some of the bitterness, or change the water out once when you cook them.

The tea is often consumed with milk and cinnamon to improve the flavor.

Medicinal Use: The astringent tannic root is the part most often used medicinally, though leaves are also used.

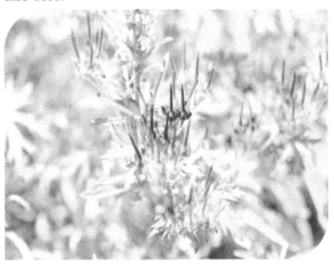

Stops Bleeding, Dries out Tissue: The entire plant is astringent and high in tannins, which causes the contraction of tissues and helps stop bleeding. Use the root or leaves as a poultice on moist wounds and for drying out tissues.

As a styptic (to stop bleeding), clean the root or leaves and apply to the wound. Hold the compress tightly for a few minutes until bleeding stops, and then bind the poultice with gauze or a clean cloth.

The plant is excellent for use in skin salves to promote skin healing.

Diarrhea and Stomach Upset: Tea made from the root is ideal for treating stomach upsets and diarrhea.

Canker Sores: Wash the canker sore with Carolina Geranium Tea or cover it with a root poultice. The astringent root is drying and reduces canker sores quickly.

Treats Sore Throats: The root is soothing for sore throats. It may have anti-viral properties as well.

Hepatitis B: Tinctured Carolina Geranium root has been shown to have the anti-Hepatitis B (HBV) compounds geraniin and hyperin.

Harvesting: Harvest young leaves and use them fresh or dry them for future use. Dig up roots in the late fall when they are plump with stored starch, or if necessary, in the early spring. Clean the roots, slice them thinly and dry for future use or use them fresh.

Recipes: Carolina Geranium Leaf Tea.
2 Tablespoons dried leaves and stems, 2 cups boiling water. Pour the boiling water over the dried leaves and allow the tea to steep, off the heat, for 10 minutes or more. Strain and enjoy.

Carolina Geranium Root Tea: The roots make the most effective medicinal tea. Bring 2 cups of water to a boil and add 2 tablespoons of chopped, dried root. Reduce the heat and simmer the tea for 10 to 15 minutes. Remove from the heat and steep for another 10 minutes. Take up to 3 cups daily.

Carolina Geranium Tincture: Sterilized glass jar with tight fitting lid, ¾ jar cleaned, chopped fresh root or ½ jar dried root, 80 proof vodka or other alcohol to fill jar.

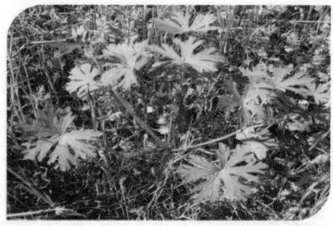

Cheese cloth or fine mesh strainer, glass bowl for straining.

Sterilize all jars, utensils, and bowls with boiling water.

Pack the jar with herbs: ¾ full for fresh root or ½ full for dried herbs, fill the jar with alcohol, making sure all herbs are covered. Cover tightly with lid.

Store the jar in a cool, dark place. Shake the jar daily for 6-8 weeks. Strain out the root and all sediment. When clean, pour into amber bottles and seal tightly. Label and date the containers

Store the bottles in a cool, dark location for up to 10 years.

Chamomile, *Matricaria chamomilla*

Chamomile is a commonly used useful herb. It is a calming plant, and has sedative properties. It is in Aster/Daisy family.

Identification: Chamomile has daisy-like flowers with a hollow, cone-shaped receptacle. Its yellow cone surrounded by 10 to 20 downward-curving white petals. You can distinguish the plant from similar flowers by the pattern in which the flowers grow, each flower on an independent stem.

The most common way of identifying chamomile is by plucking a small amount of the blossom and crushing it in between your fingers.

Chamomile has a faintly fruity scent. Chamomile grows wild and it is also easy to cultivate in the garden. It thrives in open, sunny locations with well-drained soil. It does not tolerate excessive heat or dry conditions.

Matricaria chamomilla is German chamomile. English chamomile has similar medicinal uses. The two plants can be distinguished by their leaves. German chamomile leaves are very thin and hairy while those of the English Chamomile are larger and thicker. The leaves of the German chamomile are also bipinnate; each blade can be divided again into smaller leaf sections. German chamomile stems are somewhat feathery while English Chamomile is hairless. Depending on the growing conditions chamomile can grow to between 2 feet (0.6m) and 3 feet (0.9m) tall.

Edible Use: I collect both flowers and leaves for medicinal use, but the flowers make the best tea. The flowers have an apple-like flavor, and the leaves have a grassy flavor. You can make a nice liqueur with dried chamomile flowers and vodka.

Medicinal Use: Chamomile is most often taken as a tea but it may also be taken as a tincture or as a dried encapsulated herb.

Digestive Issues: Chamomile relaxes the muscles, including the digestive muscles. This makes it a good treatment for abdominal pain, indigestion, gastritis and bloating. It is also used it for Crohn's disease and irritable bowel syndrome.

Colic: Chamomile is known to be safe for use with babies. Adding a cup of tea to the baby's bath at night soothes colic and helps with sleep.

Muscle Aches: The antispasmodic action of chamomile relieves muscle tension. It soothes aching muscles and body aches.

Insomnia: Chamomile is soothing and sedative. One cup of chamomile tea, taken at bedtime or during the night, helps with sleep. If more help is needed, use a tincture.

Eyewash, Conjunctivitis, and Pinkeye: For eye problems, try an eyewash made by dissolving 5 to 10 drops of Chamomile tincture in some boiled and cooled water or by making a strong chamomile tea.

This mixture relieves eyestrain and treats infections. I often pair it with other herbs like Yarrow and Usnea.

Asthma, Bronchitis, Whooping Cough, and Congestion: Use a steam treatment for congestion. Add two teaspoons of chamomile flower petals to a pot of boiling water. Inhale the steam until the phlegm is released. Or add 2 to 3 drops of Chamomile Essential Oil to a vaporizer and use overnight.

Allergies and Eczema: For allergic conditions, including itchy skin and eczema, try Chamomile Essential Oil. The steam distillation process alters the chemical properties of the remedy, giving it anti-allergenic properties. Dilute the essential oil in a carrier oil to use directly on the skin or inhale it.

Harvesting: It is best to harvest chamomile during its peak blooming period. I prefer to pick chamomile in

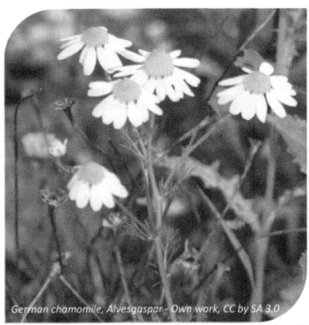

German chamomile, Alvesgaspar - Own work, CC by SA 3.0

the late morning, after the dew has evaporated and before the real heat of the day. Select flowers that are fully open and pinch or clip the flower head off at the top of the stalk. Dry for future use.

Warning: While it is uncommon, some people have an allergic reaction to chamomile. People with allergies to the Asteraceae family, including ragweed and chrysanthemums, should not take chamomile.

Recipes: Chamomile Tea. Ingredients: 1 to 2 teaspoons of dried chamomile flowers or leaves and 1 cup boiling water. Pour 1 cup of boiling water over the chamomile flowers or leaves. Let the herb steep for 5 to 10 minutes. Strain.

Chamomile Liqueur: Ingredients: 1 pint (500 ml) of 80 proof vodka, 1 cup chamomile flowers, 2 tablespoons raw honey or to taste and zest of one lemon. Combine all ingredients in a tightly covered jar and allow the mixture to steep for two to four weeks. Strain.

Chickweed, *Stellaria media*

Chickweed is an annual plant in the Caryophyllaceae (Pink) Family. This herb is naturalized to many parts of North America. It is sometimes referred to as common chickweed to distinguish it from other plants with the same name. It is also referred to as winterweed, maruns, starweed, and chickenwort among others. It is commonly grown as feed for chickens.

Identification: Common chickweed grows from 2 to 20 inches (5 cm to 50 cm) in height. Its intertwined manner of growing usually covers large areas. Its flowers are white and shaped similarly to a star. The oval leaves have cup-like tips with smooth and slightly feathered edges. Its flowers are small, white, and star-shaped. They are produced at the tip of the stem. The sepals are green in color.

Edible Use: The leaves, stem, and flowers are edible raw or cooked.

Medicinal Use. Arthritis: A tea or tincture from this herb is used as a remedy for arthritis. It relieves the inflammation and pain of rheumatoid arthritis. Also try adding a strong tea to a warm bath and soaking to relieve pain, especially on the knees and feet.

Roseola and Other Rashes: Children and adults suffering from roseola are plagued by an itchy rash. Use a poultice of moistened crushed chickweed leaves applied to the rash for relief of pain and itching. Adding a strong tea to the bathwater also helps.

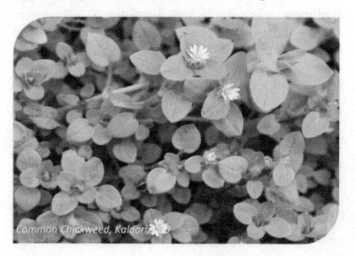
Common Chickweed, Kaldari

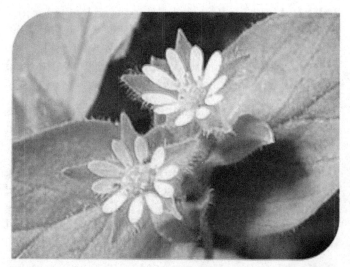

Nerve Pain: Chickweed applied as a poultice or salve helps relieve the pain and tingling caused by surface nerves misfiring.

Constipation and Digestive Problems: Chickweed tea treats constipation. Be careful not to overdo it with the decoction; it has a strong purgative action.

Chickweed also has analgesic properties that act on the digestive system to relieve pain, but it does not treat the underlying causes.

Skin Irritations, Dermatitis, Eczema, Hives, Shingles, and Varicose Veins: A salve or poultice made from chickweed works well for skin irritations, especially on itches and rashes. It is also useful for varicose veins, hives, dermatitis, and eczema. You can add the decoction to your bath if the affected area is larger.

Detoxification, Blood Purification, Tetanus, Boils, Herpes, and Venereal Diseases: Chickweed is an excellent detoxification agent and blood purifier. It draws poisons out of the body in cases of blood poisoning, tetanus, or from poisons entering the bloodstream through a wound.

For these purposes make a poultice from equal parts chickweed, ginger root, and raw honey. Blend the mixture to a smooth paste and apply it directly to the wound and the surrounding area.

Cover the poultice and replace it every six hours. Also take chickweed powder or tea to treat the problem from the inside out. This same protocol works for the treatment of boils, herpes sores, and other venereal diseases. Take both internal and external remedies for best results.

Harvesting: Harvest this herb early in the morning or late in the evening. Snip off the upper branches. Use them fresh or dry them for future use.

Warning: Some people are allergic to chickweed. The herb is considered safe, but should not be used by nursing women or pregnant women without the approval from a healthcare professional.

Recipes. Chickweed Decoction: Use fresh chickweed whenever possible to make this herbal decoction. It is an excellent internal cleanser and makes a good wash and external agent. You need 1 cup freshly picked chickweed leaves and 1 pint (500 ml) of water. Bring the water to a boil and add the chickweed leaves. Reduce the heat to low and simmer the leaves for 15 minutes. Cool the decoction and use it internally or externally. The internal dose is 1 to 2 ounces (30 to 60ml).

Chicory,
Cichorium intybus

Common chicory is an annual or biannual plant in the Aster/Daisy Family. It originated from Eurasia and is found throughout North America, where it is known as an invasive species in several places. Common chicory is also called blue daisy, blue dandelion, blue sailors, blue weed, coffeeweed, cornflower, succory, wild bachelor's buttons, wild endive, and horseweed.

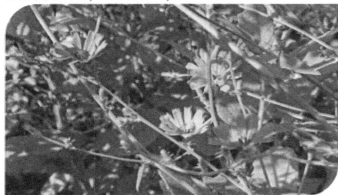

It is sometimes confused with Curly Endive (*Cichorium endivia*), a closely related plant often called chicory.

Identification: Chicory is easy to identify by its purple flowers when in bloom. Its stems are rigid with hairy lower stems. Its alternate lobed leaves are coarsely toothed and similar to dandelion leaves in appearance. The lower leaves are covered with hairs and grow up to 8 inches (20 cm) in length. The stems and leaves both exude a milky latex when cut.

The plant grows 1 to 3 feet (0.3m to 0.9m) tall and has numerous flower heads, each around 1 to 1 1/2 inches (2.5 cm to 3.75 cm) wide, appearing in clusters of two or three. Light blue-purple (and rarely pink or white)

flowers bloom from July thru October. Petals grow in two rows with toothed ends. The blooms are open in the morning but close during the heat of the day. Its root is a thick, fleshy bitter taproot.

Edible Use: The leaves have a bitter taste, which can be reduced by boiling and draining. I prefer young leaves boiled, then sautéed with garlic and butter. The most famous use of chicory is as a coffee additive or substitute. Roast the roots and grind them. Roots may be eaten raw or cooked.

Medicinal Use: Chicory roots and seeds help eliminate intestinal worms and parasites, are antibacterial, antifungal, and hepatoprotective. Roots are being studied for use in cancer. The flowers and leaves are also used medicinally. It is a mild diuretic.

Sedative and Analgesic: The milky juice from the fresh root of chicory is similar to the milky sap of Wild Lettuce (*Lactuca* spp.), also in this book. They contain lactucin and lactucopicrin, which are sedative and analgesic (pain-killing). They are sesquiterpene lactones, so it is recommended to use the latex as is or, if you want a liquid form, to dry them and then extract the medicine in high proof alcohol or oil versus in water. Pain-relief is similar to ibuprofen.

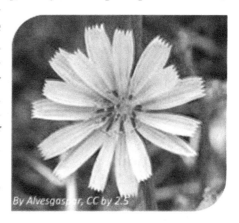
By Alvesgaspar, CC by 2.5

Antibacterial and Anti-Fungal (*Candida*): Chicory seed and root extracts are antibacterial and anti-fungal. Seeds work against *Staphylococcus*,

Pseudomonas, E. coli, and *Candida*. Roots work to kill *Staphylococcus, Bacillus, Salmonella, E. coli*, and *Micrococcus* as well as athlete's foot, ringworm, and jock itch. It can be taken internally and externally.

Anti-Parasitic and Malaria: Chicory root alcoholic extractions eliminate intestinal worms and the protozoan responsible for cerebral malaria (Plasmodium falciparum). The roots contain lactucin and lactucopicrin, both anti-malarials.

Liver and Gallbladder Disorders: The leaves, seeds, and roots of chicory are used to treat liver disorders. They are hepatoprotective. They promote the secretion of bile, treat jaundice, and treat enlargement of the spleen. They help fatty liver and to detox the liver.

Diabetes: Chicory leaf tincture, leaf powder, or a whole-plant alcoholic extraction helps regulate insulin levels, stimulate insulin secretion, and lower blood glucose levels.

Digestive Problems and Ulcers: Chicory coffee or tea made from the roots helps treat digestive problems and ulcers.

Skin Eruptions, Swellings, and Inflammations: For external use, wash blemishes with a chicory leaf infusion or apply crushed leaves as a poultice to areas of inflammation. Many people report that chicory infusion used as a wash nourishes the skin and gives it a more radiant and youthful appearance. It can be used as a face and body wash daily.

Harvesting: Only harvest plants that have not been exposed to car fumes and chemical spray along roadsides.

Leaves and flowers are easily picked throughout the season. Harvest the roots in the late autumn. Loosen the soil around the base of each plant, grab the plant at the base, and pull up as much of the tap root as possible. Clean and use them fresh or cut and dry them for future use.

Warning: Chicory can cause contact dermatitis in some people. It also causes skin irritations and rashes in some people if taken internally. Avoid chicory during pregnancy; it can stimulate menstruation. Chicory can interfere with beta-blocker drugs for the heart.

Recipes. Chicory Coffee: Clean the roots and chop them into small pieces. Lay them out on a cookie sheet to roast. Roast them in a very slow oven or over a fire. When the roots are completely roasted and dried throughout, grind them into a powder. Store the powder sealed in a cool, dry place. Brew like you would coffee.

Chives, Allium schoenoprasum

Allium schoenoprasum belongs to the Amaryllidaceae (Amaryllis) Family. It is a close relative of garlics, shallots, and leeks. These herbs are often cultivated in home gardens, but also occur wild in many areas. They are widespread across North America, Europe, and Asia. They are mostly used as a culinary herb.

Identification: Chives are bulb-forming plants that grow from 12 to 20 inches (30 cm to 50 cm) tall. Their slender bulbs are about an inch (2.5 cm) long and nearly 1/2 inch (1.25 cm) across. They grow from roots in dense clusters. The stems are tubular and hollow and grow up to 20 inches (50 cm) long and about an inch across. The stems have a softer texture before the emergence of the flower. Chives have grass-like leaves, which are shorter than the stems. The leaves are also tubular or round in cross-section and are hollow, which distinguishes it from garlic chives, *Allium tuberosum*.

Chives usually flower in April to May in southern regions and in June in northern regions. Its flowers are usually pale purple and grow in a dense inflorescence of 10 to 30 flowers that is 1/2 to 1 inch (1.25 cm to 2.5 cm) wide. Before opening, the inflorescence is typically surrounded by a papery bract. Fruits are small, 3-sectioned capsules. The seeds mature in the summer.

Edible Use: The leaves, roots, and flowers are all edible. Leaves have a mild onion flavor.

Medicinal Use: Chives have similar medical properties to those of garlic but are weaker overall. For this reason, it is used to a limited extent as a medicinal herb. Chives are also a mild stimulant, and have antiseptic and diuretic properties.

Digestion: Chives contain sulfide compounds, antibacterial compounds, and antifungal compounds that are effective in easing digestion and an upset stomach. They also stimulate the appetite.

Lowers Blood Pressure, Cholesterol, and Promotes Heart Health: Like other plants in the onion family, chives contain allicin, which helps reduce the levels of bad cholesterol in the body and improves the circulatory system and heart health. Regular consumption of chives reduces arterial plaques, relaxes the blood vessels, lowers high blood pressure, and decreases the risk of heart attacks and strokes.

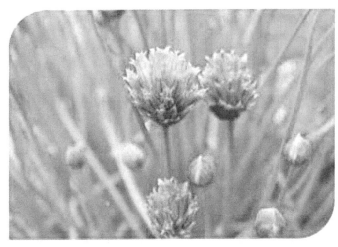

Anti-inflammatory: Chives have mild anti-inflammatory properties and are a good addition to the diet for people with diseases that involve inflammation, such as arthritis, autoimmune conditions, and inflammatory skin conditions.

Boosts the Immune System: Chives contain a wide range of vitamins and minerals, including vitamin C, which helps boost the immune system and stimulates the production of white blood cells.

Harvesting: Chives can be harvested as soon as they are big enough to clip and use. Snip off the leaves at the base. The plant will continue to grow and can be harvested 3 to 4 times a year when young (the first year) and even monthly as they mature. Store them fresh in the refrigerator or dry them for future use.

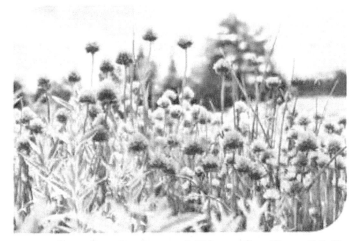

Detoxing the Body and Diuretic: The mild diuretic properties of chives help flush toxins from the body and encourage urination.

Comfrey, *Symphytum officinale*

Comfrey, is a member of the borage family. The herb is easily grown in your home garden and grows like a weed in many areas. It is also known as knit bone, boneset and slippery root.

Identification: Comfrey is a vigorous perennial herb with long lance-like leaves, each 12 to 18 inches (30 cm to 45 cm) long. The hairy leaves grow from a central crown on the ends of short stems. The plant reaches 2 to 5 feet (0.6m to 1.5m) in height and spreads to over 3 feet (0.9m) in diameter. It can be propagated from cuttings but is not invasive once planted. Comfrey flowers begin as a blue to purple bell, fading to pink as

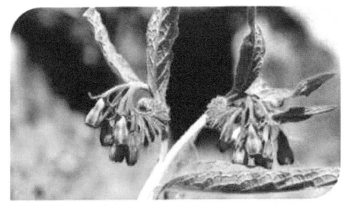

they age. The thick, tuberous roots have a thin black skin.

Edible Use: Comfrey leaves and roots are not edible because they contain small amounts of toxins that should not be consumed. The leaves can be used to make a medicinal tea or gargle.

Medicinal Use: This herb is a valuable remedy that accelerates healing of the skin and wounds. A compress of the roots or leaves can be applied directly to the skin or made into a salve. It inhibits the growth of bacteria, helping to prevent infections, and minimizes scarring. It is mucilaginous and contains the compound allantoin, which boosts cell growth and repair. It also is an excellent anti-inflammatory and relieves pain, inflammation, and swelling in joints and muscles. Comfrey tea is best used to alleviate stomach problems, heavy menstrual bleeding, bloody urine, breathing problems, cancer, and chest pain. Be careful with internal use (see Warning section). It can also be gargled to treat gum disease or sore throat.

Sprains, Bruises and Breaks: Comfrey Salve or comfrey compresses are one of the best remedies for sprains, strains, bruised muscles and joints, and fractured bones. The herb speeds up healing while increasing mobility and relieving the pain and swelling. Apply the salvet or a poultice made from crushed comfrey root up to four times a day. Make sure that a broken bone is set before applying comfrey.

Back Pain: Use comfrey root salve to treat back pain. Applied three times a day, it relieves bone and joint pains.

Osteoarthritis: Likewise, external Comfrey Salve is beneficial for knee and joint pain due to osteoarthritis.

Coughs, Congestion, and Asthma: Comfrey Tea treats coughs, congestion, and asthma. The herb reduces the inflammation and soothes the irritation.

Minor Skin Injuries, Burns, Rashes, Eczema, Psoriasis and Wounds: One of the best uses for comfrey is in healing minor injuries to the skin. Rashes, eczema, burns, and skin wounds heal quickly when the herb is used. I prefer to use the root for this purpose, but leaves can also be used. Apply Comfrey Salve three times a day or use bruised leaves or crushed root to make a poultice for the damaged skin. I also use Comfrey Tea or Comfrey Root Decoction as a wash for the area, especially for rashes, acne, eczema, and psoriasis. Do not use for deep wounds or puncture wounds as it heals them too quickly, blocking in infection.

Stomach Upsets, Ulcers of the Stomach and Lungs: Comfrey is used to treat internal ulcers and the bleeding they cause. The comfrey stops the bleeding and helps the wounded tissue heal. You can drink the tea or use the decoction.

Harvesting: Comfrey leaves are best harvested in the spring or early summer, before the plant blooms. They can be harvested in several cuttings and dried for later use. The roots can be dug at any time as needed. Leave behind part of the roots to encourage continued growth and an additional crop the next year.

Warning: Harmful toxins in comfrey are believed to cause liver damage, lung damage, or cancer when used in highly concentrated doses. For this reason, many healers do not recommend internal use of comfrey. However, small doses have been used safely in herbal medicines for hundreds of years with no reported ill effects. Use internally with caution or under care.

Comfrey should not be used by pregnant or breastfeeding women.

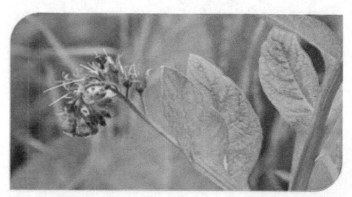

Both oral use and skin application could be hazardous and could cause birth defects. Do not use comfrey if you have liver disease or any liver problems. Comfrey heals wounds very quickly. As such, it is recommended that bone fractures and bone breaks are properly set before using it. This also applies for puncture wounds, as its rapid healing can seal in the bacterial infection.

Recipes. Comfrey Salve.: You'll need: Comfrey root and/or leaves to fill a pint (500ml) jar, 1 cup Organic Olive Oil and 1/4 cup of beeswax, or more.

Allow the comfrey leaves and root to dry, removing excess moisture. This can be done in a low oven, dehydrator, or by leaving them out in a warm place for a few days. Turn the oven on to its lowest setting.

Place the dried leaves and chopped root pieces into a pint (500ml) jar. Add 1 cup of olive oil and place the open jar in the oven. Allow the oil to warm and infuse for 90 minutes. Remove the jar from the oven and cover with a cloth to cool. When cool, place the lid on the jar and allow it to steep for 2 to 3 weeks in a cool, dark place. Strain the oil, removing the leaves and roots.

Combine the oil and the beeswax in a pot and warm gently until the beeswax is melted (4:1 ratio of oil to beeswax). Test the consistency of the oil by dipping a small amount onto waxed paper or aluminum foil and place in the freezer for five minutes. If the oil is thick enough, pour the mixture into a jar or wide mouth container. If not add a little more beeswax and test again.

Continue until desired consistency is reached. If the mixture is too thick you can warm it again and stir in a little more oil. Note: use an old non-aluminum pot to heat the oil and wax. It is difficult to clean. I have a small pot that I use only for this purpose.

Common Flax, *Linum usitatissimum*

Also known as Linseed, this is a useful plant for making medicine, oil, and fabric. Many people take it as a nutritional supplement. It is in the *Linaceae* (Flax) Family.

Identification: Common Flax is an annual. While rarely found growing wild, it is usually easy to find a cultivated crop or to grow yourself. The mature plant is 3 to 4 feet (0.9m to 1.2m) tall. A loose cluster of blue-purple stalked flowers grows at the tips of the branching stems. Each ¾ to 1 inch (2 cm to 2.5 cm) wide flower has 5 ovate petals surrounded by 5 erect, blue-tipped stamens with a green ovary. The 5 sepals have a lance-shape. Flax has simple, alternate, erect green leaves that are 1/2 to 1 1/2 inches (1.25 cm to 3.75 cm) long and very narrow. They are stalkless and have smooth margins. Its stems are mostly unbranched and erect, and has multiple round, smooth stems growing from its base. Flax fruit is a round, dry, 5-lobed capsule that is 1/4 -1/2 (0.75 cm to 1.25 cm) inch in diameter.

Edible Use: The sprouts and seeds can be eaten raw or cooked. Careful eating the sprouts raw as they can stop up the bowel. Chew seeds well to access their nutrition, as they don't digest well whole.

Medicinal Use. As a Nutritional Supplement: Flax seed is rich in dietary fiber, protein, omega-3 fatty acids, and other nutrients. I grind flax and chia seeds fresh and eat them daily for health. I find that the fresh seeds are better as oil goes rancid quite quickly.

Cholesterol Control: Ingesting crushed flaxseeds on a daily basis is a good way to lower your cholesterol and LDL.

Autoimmune Issues: Flax seeds are high in omega 3 fatty acids, alpha-linolenic acid (ALA), and lignans. These compounds help regulate immune response, suppress inflammation, have neuroprotective effects, act as antioxidants, and modulate hormonal influences in autoimmune conditions.

Respiratory Problems: Flax seed oil helps with respiratory problems, including ARDS (acute respiratory distress syndrome). Its anti-inflammatory effects help coughs, sore throat, and congestion.

Constipation: For constipation, try two teaspoons of ground flax seed every morning, taken with a full glass of water.

Skin, Boils, Abscesses, Herpes, Acne, Burns: A warm poultice of flax seed oil on a cotton ball or applied directly helps heal these common skin problems. Flax is an excellent anti-inflammatory both internally and externally. For boils, add *Lobelia inflata*

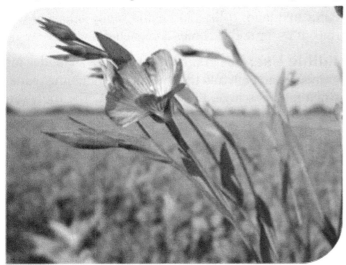

root to flax seed oil and apply it directly to the boil or use as a poultice.

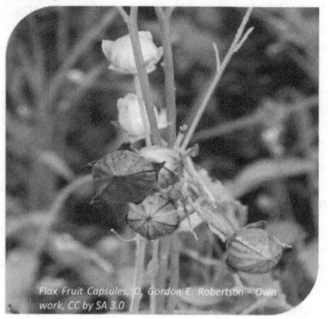

Flax Fruit Capsules, D. Gordon E. Robertson - Own work, CC by SA 3.0

Balancing Hormones: Flax seed contains lignans, a type of phytoestrogen. This helps balance female hormones, especially in post-menopausal women, and helps with symptoms of menopause.

Cancer: Flax seed and flax seed oil work as a complementary treatment as well as for the prevention of breast cancer and prostate cancer, where they seem to reduce PSA (prostate specific antigen) levels. Flax seeds help decrease breast cancer risk, lower the risk of metastasizing, and help to kill cancer cells in post-menopausal women. Consult with your oncologist.

Harvesting: Flax seed is harvested in the same manner as wheat. Harvest when the plant and fruits are dry and the seedpods begin to split. Shake over a sheet and sift. You may have to crush the seedpods to access the seeds.

Warning and Recommendations: Ground and powdered flax seed go rancid very quickly. I keep my flax seed whole until I need them, then grind or crush only the needed amount. Drink plenty of water with flax seeds.

Couch Grass, *Agropyron (Elymus) repens*

Couch Grass is often considered a simple weed and a nuisance; however, it has a list of medicinal properties that can't be ignored. It is also called dog grass, witchgrass, quack grass, and twitch grass. It can grow up to 3 feet (0.9m) tall and is part of the Poaceae (Grass) Family.

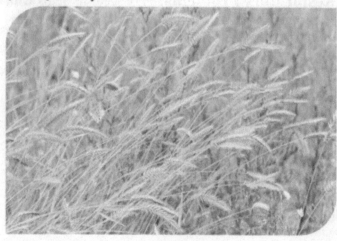

Identification: The crawling tubular root is elongated while the leaves are slender. Each short stem produces five to seven leaves and possibly a flower spike at the terminal. Each flower spike is composed of oval-shaped spikelets less than an inch (2.5 cm) long. The flowers appear in late June through August. The seed heads look like a stalk of grain. The roots are elongated, thin, tubular and whitish in color with yellow ends. Couch grass grows aggressively and is capable of crowding out agricultural crops and is often found on cultivated land. It likes loose and sandy soils and will die out as the soil becomes compacted.

Edible Use: The grain has food value as fodder for animals, and I am told that the root is sometimes eaten when food is scarce. I've never tried it. The roots can also be ground and roasted to make a coffee substitute.

Medicinal Use: Use the rhizomes of this plant to make a tincture, infusion, or decoction.

Urinary Tract Problems, Kidney Stones, Cystitis, Gallbladder Diseases: Couch grass is effective at treating urinary tract problems including inflammations, infections, and slow and painful urination caused by muscle spasms of the bladder and urethra. It soothes the mucous membranes and relieves the pain. It is a diuretic that increases the production of urine. It also works to dissolve kidney stones and gravel and treat cystitis and diseases of the gallbladder. Try using couch grass in combination with Usnea and bearberry to treat urinary tract infections.

Swollen Prostate: The herb is effective for treatment of swollen prostate glands, especially from gonorrhea. It is often combined with saw palmetto for this use.

Gout: Try couch grass decoction for treating gout.

Rheumatoid Arthritis: The diuretic properties, anti-inflammatory properties, and analgesic properties of couch grass make it effective in treating rheumatoid arthritis.

Jaundice: The anti-inflammatory properties and diuretic properties, combined with the benefits to the urinary tract and gallbladder, make couch grass a good choice for treating jaundice. It helps the body eliminate toxins and allows it to heal.

Recipes. Couch Grass Decoction: Ingredients: 4 ounces (113g) couch grass roots, chopped and 1-quart (1 Liter) water. Bring the water and the roots to a boil and reduce the heat to a simmer. Simmer the roots, uncovered, until the liquid is reduced by half, leaving approximately 2 cups of liquid. Store in the refrigerator for 3 days or freeze for longer periods.

Dandelion, *Taraxacum officinale*

Most children relish the opportunity to blow a puff of dandelion seeds into the wind. This wonderful plant is commonly regarded as a weed and can be found growing in sidewalk cracks and across untended roadsides and lawns. There are some look-alike flowers, so be sure of your identification before harvesting the plant. It is in the Aster/Daisy Family.

Identification: Dandelion is a perennial herbaceous plant native to North America. It grows from a tap-root that reaches deep into the soil. The plant grows up to a foot in height and flowers from April to June. It produces a yellow flower head consisting of florets. Leaves grow from the base of the plant in an elongated shape with highly jagged edges. The edges are said to resemble a lion's tooth, giving the plant its name.

Edible Use: The entire plant is edible and nutritious. The young leaves are best for greens, since the leaves grow more bitter with age. Young leaves can be cooked or eaten raw. Dandelion root is sometimes dried and roasted for use as a coffee substitute. The roots can also be cooked and eaten. They are bitter, with a taste similar to a turnip. Dandelion flowers make a nice salad garnish or can be battered and fried. Unopened flower buds are prepared into pickles similar to capers. Flowers can also be boiled and served with butter. Dandelion leaves and roots make a pleasant, but bitter tea. Flowers are fermented to make

dandelion wine. Leaves and roots are used to flavor herbal beers and soft drinks.

Medicinal Use: The entire dandelion plant is used medicinally. The bitter roots are good for gastrointestinal and liver problems, while the leaves have a powerful diuretic effect. The plant makes a great general tonic and benefits the entire body. It is high in vitamins, minerals, and antioxidants. I use dandelion tea and tincture for internal use.

Digestion Problems, Liver and Gallbladder Function: Dandelion root is used to aid digestion and benefits the kidneys, gallbladder, and liver. It stimulates bile production, helping with the digestion of fats and toxin removal. Use it to treat jaundice and raise energy levels after infections. It removes toxins from the body and restores the electrolyte balance, which improves liver health and function.

I do a 2-week liver cleanse with my homemade Liver Tonic – a Dandelion Root and Milk Thistle seed tincture blend – every 6 months for general health. It also helps prevent gallstones. Dandelion contains inulin, a carbohydrate that helps maintain healthy gut flora and helps to regulate blood sugar levels. The plant is rich in fiber, which adds bulk to the stool, reducing the

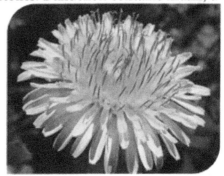

Dandelion FlowerGreg Hume, CC BY-SA 3.0

chances of constipation, diarrhea, and digestive issues.

Liver Protection and Healing: Vitamins and antioxidants in dandelion protect the liver and keep it healthy. It helps protect the liver from toxins and treats liver hemorrhages. Dandelion tea is used to treat non-alcoholic fatty liver disease. My Liver Tonic Blend (Dandelion Root and Milk Thistle Seed extract) reversed a patient's liver disease to the point that she no longer needs a liver transplant. This blend is also good for cirrhosis and hepatitis.

Diuretic and Detoxifying the Body: Dandelion leaves are a powerful diuretic and blood purifier. They stimulate the liver and gallbladder while eliminating toxins through the production and excretion of urine. They also help flush the kidneys. Even though dandelion is a diuretic it helps replace lost potassium and other minerals that are lost when water and salts are expelled.

Skin Wounds, Corns, and Warts: Fresh dandelion juice applied to the skin helps wounds heal and fights the bacteria and fungi that would otherwise cause infections. Dandelion sap, sometimes called dandelion milk, is useful to treat itches, ringworm, eczema, warts, and corns. Apply dandelion sap directly to the affected skin. Dandelion tea can be used as a wash on the skin to help healing. Dandelion sap is also useful in treating acne. It inhibits the formation of acne blemishes and reduces scarring. Some people are allergic to dandelion sap, so watch for signs of dermatitis on first use.

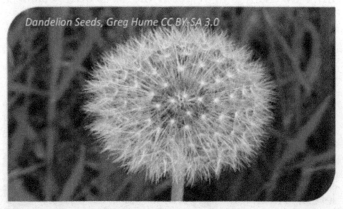

Dandelion Seeds, Greg Hume CC BY-SA 3.0

Osteoporosis and Bone Health: The calcium and vitamin K found in dandelion can protect bones from osteoporosis and arthritis. It helps stabilize bone density and strengthen the bone.

Controls Blood Sugar: Dandelion has several effects that are beneficial to diabetics. Dandelion juice stimulates the production of insulin in the pancreas, which helps regulate blood sugar levels and prevent dangers blood sugar swings. The plant is a natural diuretic which helps remove excess sugars from the body. It also helps control lipid levels.

Urinary Tract Disorders: The diuretic nature of dandelion helps eliminate toxins from the kidneys and urinary tract. The herb also acts as a disinfectant, inhibiting bacterial growth in the urinary system.

Prevents and Treats Cancer: Dandelion extracts are high in antioxidants, which reduce free radicals in the body and the risk of cancer. Its role in removing toxins from the body is also helpful. Researchers have shown that Dandelion Root coupled with Burdock Root have potential in treating cancer.

Prevents Iron Deficiency Anemia: Dandelions have high levels of iron, vitamins, and other minerals. Iron is an important part of the hemoglobin in blood and essential for healthy red blood cell formation. Using dandelion and eating the greens helps keep iron levels high.

Treating Hypertension: As a diuretic, dandelion juice helps eliminate excess sodium from the body and bring down blood pressure. It also helps reduce cholesterol ratios and raises the "good" HDL levels.

Boosts the Immune System: Dandelion boosts the immune system and helps fight off microbial and fungal agents.

Mastitis and Lactation: Dandelion has traditionally been used to enhance milk production and for treatment of mastitis. Check in with your doctor for this use.

Fights Inflammation and Arthritis: Dandelion contains antioxidants, phytonutrients and essential fatty acids that reduce inflammation in the body. This relieves swelling and related pain in the body. Inflammation is the root cause of many diseases, such as arthritis. Taraxasterol, found in dandelion roots, has shown great promise for Osteoarthritis.

Harvesting: I prefer to gather dandelion leaves in the spring when they are young and less bitter. I dry them for later medicinal use. Often, they grow in lawns or parks that have been sprayed so be careful where you harvest them.

For roots, I prefer the roots of plants that are 2-years old or older. The roots are larger and more medicinally potent. Grab the plant at the base and pull the entire plant up. The root is a deep taproot and will require some force.

You can also dig around the plant at a modest distance to help remove the entire root. As many gardeners know, leaving just a bit of the root will allow the plant to regrow.

So, if you want more dandelions simply leave part of the root intact. Plants dug in the autumn have more medicinal properties and higher levels of inulin.

Warning: Dandelion is generally considered safe, although some people may be allergic to it. Do not take dandelion if you are allergic to plants from the same family, or similar plants such as ragweed, chrysanthemum, marigold, yarrow, or daisy. Do not take dandelion if you are pregnant and consult your doctor if nursing.

Consult your doctor before taking if you are taking prescription medicines. Some people have reported dermatitis as a result of touching the plant or using the sap. Do not use dandelion if you are allergic.

Recipes: Dandelion Tea. Ingredients: 1/2 to 2 teaspoons of roasted dandelion root, in small pieces and 1 cup of boiling water. Pour boiling water over roasted or dried dandelion root and allow it to steep for 20 minutes. Strain the tea and drink.

Do not add sweeteners, as they reduce the herb's effectiveness. Milk may be used to taste, if desired.

Drink 3 cups per day for general medicinal use.

Dill,
Anethum graveolens

Dill is a familiar aromatic herb cultivated in herb gardens across the country. It is in the Apiaceae /Umbelliferae (Celery/Carrot) Family.

Identification: Dill grows to 30 inches (75 cm) tall with a slender, hollow, and erect stem and feathery leaves. Leaves are finely divided and delicate in appearance, and are 4 to 8 inches (10 cm to 20 cm) long. They are similar to fennel in appearance.

Numerous tiny yellow or white flowers appear on umbrellas that are 3/4 to 3 1/2 inches (1.875 cm to 8.75 cm) in diameter as soon as the weather turns hot.

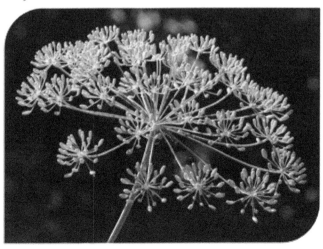

The seeds are small, up to 1/5 of an inch (0.625 cm) long with a ridged surface.

Edible Use: Dill is widely enjoyed as an herb, especially with fish and in pickles. The leaves, seeds, and stems are edible.

Medicinal Use. Colic: Colicky babies respond well to a dill infusion. The dill soothes the stomach and calms the baby. This is a popular colic remedy because it is easily attained, effective, and known to be safe for children.

Digestive Issues, Irritable Bowel Syndrome, Menstrual Cramps, and Muscle Spasms: Dill Leaf Infusion relieves cramping and muscle spasms including those in the digestive tract. It relieves the symptoms of painful spasms without treating the underlying cause. Use it to give immediate relief while looking for the cause of the problem. A Dill Seed Infusion or Dill Tincture may also be used.

Stimulates Milk Flow: Dill Infusion helps nursing mothers increase their milk flow. It has a beneficial calming effect on both mother and child.

Halitosis: Temporary bad breath is easily solved by chewing on dill leaves or seeds, but the problem can be completely alleviated by chewing the seeds daily. Over the long term the seeds attack the causes of the problem causing a permanent solution.

Flatulence: For abdominal flatulence, take Dill Seed Infusion before each meal.

Harvesting: Harvest leaves throughout the summer until the flowers appear in late summer. Gather leaves in the late morning after the dew has dried and use them fresh, freeze them, or dry them for later use. I collect the seed heads once the flowers are fully open, if needed, or I allow them to completely ripen for seed collection. The brown seeds are collected and dried for storage.

Warning: Consumption of dill can cause sensitivity to the sun in some people. People sometimes have a rash appear after exposure to sunlight.

Recipes. Dill Leaf Infusion: Ingredients: 1 Tablespoon chopped dill leaves and 1 cup boiling water. Pour the boiling water over the dill leaves and cover the cup.

Let it steep until cool enough to drink, then strain out the leaves.

Dill Seed Infusion: You need 1 to 2 tablespoons dill seeds and 1 cup water. Bring the seeds and water to a boil, turn off the heat and cover the pot. Allow the infusion to steep for 15 minutes. Cool and strain out the seeds. Take one cup before each meal for digestive issues.

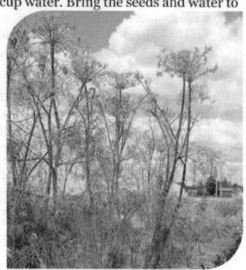

Dock (Curly/Yellow), *Rumex crispus*

Docks and Sorrels, genus *Rumex*, is a group of over 200 different varieties in the Polygonaceae (Buckwheat) Family. Here I am referring specifically to *Rumex crispus* and its medicinal use, but broad-leaved dock, *Rumex obstusifolius*, is used in a similar manner. Curly Dock is a biennial herb that grows across the globe. The plant is also called yellow dock, sour dock, narrow-leaved dock, and curled dock.

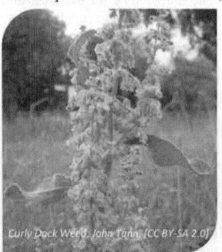

Curly Dock Weed, John Tann, [CC BY-SA 2.0]

Identification: Flower stalks grow from the base (similar to a rosette) with smooth, leathery, fleshy leaves growing in a large cluster at the apex. Leaves are wavy or curly on the edges and have a coarse texture. These leaves can grow up to 2 feet (0.6m) long and are only 3 inches (7.5 cm) wide, making them long, narrow

and wavy. Small veins curve out toward the edge of the leaf and then turn back towards the central vein. Leaves farther up the plant may vary in size and appearance. On older leaves the central vein is sometimes tinged with red.

The flower stalk is approximately 3 feet (0.9m) in height with clustered flowers and seeds. Tiny green flowers grow in dense heads on the flower stalk during the second year.

The 3-sided seeds are brown, shiny, and covered by a papery sheath that looks like heart-shaped wings. The root is a long yellow, forking taproot that regenerates the plant each year.

Edible Use: Curly dock has a lemony flavor and its leaves are used as a cooked vegetable. Young leaves can

1Curly Dock Weed, By Olivier Pichard [CC BY-SA 3.0]

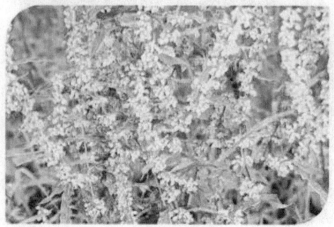

be eaten raw (old ones can too but they don't taste as good). Leaves contain varying amounts of oxalic acid and tannin. The seeds can be pounded into a flour. The root is generally not eaten but it is used for medicine.

Medicinal Use: Curly dock is a purifying and cleansing herb. All parts of the plant can be used, but the roots have the strongest healing properties.

I often crush dock leaves to put on stinging nettle stings. My grandmother showed me this trick when I was a child visiting her in England and I've been using it ever since. They tend to grow near each other, which is very useful.

Constipation and Diarrhea: Curly dock is a gentle and safe laxative for the treatment of mild constipation. It can also cause or relieve diarrhea, depending on the dosage and other factors such as harvest time and soil conditions.

Skin Problems: Curly dock weed is useful externally to treat a wide variety of skin problems due to its cleansing properties.

Taken internally, it is a tonic. Its dried or pounded root can be used as a poultice, salve, or powder applied to sores, wounds, or other skin problems.

Liver, Gall Bladder and Detox: Curly dock root is a bitter tonic for the gall bladder and liver. It increases bile production, which helps the body with detoxification. It is helpful for any condition that can benefit from purifying and cleansing the body from toxins. It is often combined with Greater Burdock to create a stronger detoxifying effect.

Harvesting: Harvest the root early in autumn and dry it for later use. Dig up the entire plant and root if possible and wash the root lightly. Cut before drying. Harvest leaves from spring through summer as needed. Look for leaves that are fresh and curled. Avoid leaves that are brown or full of bug holes. Also avoid areas that are near highways or that have been sprayed with pesticides.

Recipes. Curly Dock Tincture: You need fresh curly dock root, grated, 80-proof vodka or other drinking alcohol and a glass jar with tight-fitting lid. Place the grated root in a clean glass jar. Fill the jar, covering the root completely, with 80-proof alcohol.

Allow the tincture to steep for 6 to 8 weeks, shaking gently every day. Strain out the root pieces and place the tincture in a clean glass jar. Store in a cool, dark place for up to 7 years.

Echinacea angustifolia and *E. purpurea*, Purple Coneflower

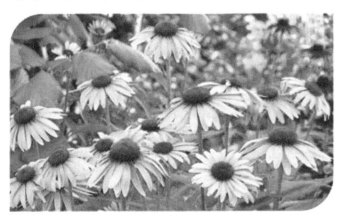
Close up of flower disc, Photo by Bernie, CC by SA 3.0

Echinacea is commonly called Purple Coneflower. It is a pretty, purple sunflower-like flowering plant that has strong medicine. It is native to North America and belongs to the Asteraceae (Daisy) Family. It is widespread and easy to cultivate in the garden. Echinacea grows wild in open rocky prairies and plains.

Identification: Purple coneflower is a perennial herb that is 6 to 24 inches (15 cm to 60 cm) tall with a woody, often branching taproot. This plant has one to several rough-hairy stems that are mostly unbranched.

The leaves are alternate, simple, and narrowly lance-shaped. The stem leaves are widely spaced and attached alternately to the lower half of the stem. Edges of leaves are toothless and have three distinct veins along its length. Stem and leaves are rough and hairy to touch. Its stems may be purple or green tinged. Echinacea Flowers look like lavender sunflowers. Its flowerheads are 1 ½ to 3 inches (3.75 cm to 7.5 cm) wide and are at the ends of long stalks. They bloom in summer. The disk flowers are 5-lobed, brownish-purple in color, and are situated among stiff bracts with yellow pollen. Its fruits are small, dark, 4- angled achenes.

Medicinal Use: This herb has a modulating effect on the body's natural immune system, encouraging it

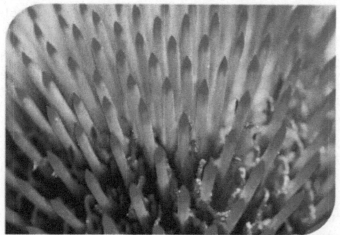

For Infections, Burns, Wounds and as an Anti-Fungal: Echinacea is an antibiotic, antifungal antiviral, and it stimulates the immune system. It is helpful to relieve infections of all kinds. It is used both externally and internally.

Snakebite, Insect and Spider Bites, and Stings: Echinacea is used to treat spider bites and insect stings. It does a good job of neutralizing the poison and reducing the pain. It is said to be useful for snakebites, as it is a strong anti-inflammatory.

Harvesting: Harvest the roots in autumn when the plant has died back. Dig up the entire plant, watching for branched roots. Scrub the dirt from the root and dry it for later use.

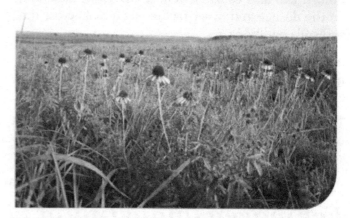

to operate more efficiently. It raises the body's resistance to bacterial and viral infections by stimulating the immune system. It also has anti-inflammatory and pain-relieving functions.

Do not use internally if you have an autoimmune condition. Most people seem aware that Echinacea is an herb for preventing and healing colds and the flu, but these plants can do a lot more. The root and leaves are used medicinally.

Urinary Tract Infections: The anti-microbial and anti-inflammatory effects of Echinacea make it an ideal choice for the treatment of urinary tract infections. It is a standard UTI treatment and is often combined with goldenseal root. Do not take either of these herbs if you have an autoimmune condition.

Colds and the Flu: Echinacea is known to reduce the impact of the common cold and the flu. People who begin taking Echinacea extract or tea immediately upon feeling sick heal much more quickly than those who do not.

In general, people who take Echinacea get well up to 4 days faster than those who don't (note that the same holds true for blue elderberry). For best results, they should begin taking Echinacea as soon as they notice symptoms, taking a double dose three times on the first day and then take three regular doses each day during the illness.

Allergies and Respiratory Diseases: Echinacea helps to relieve allergies by stimulating and balancing the immune system. It is especially helpful in relieving asthma attacks. While it doesn't cure asthma, it reduces the severity of the attack and helps the patient get over attacks. It is also useful for treating bronchitis.

Warning: Do not use internally long-tem as it may cause digestive upset. People with autoimmune conditions should not use Echinacea internally as it is an immune-system booster and may lead to a flare-up.

Recipes. Echinacea Tincture: 1-pint (500ml) of vodka or rum, at least 80 proof, 1 cup of loosely packed Echinacea leaf and root, chopped fine, 1-pint(500ml) glass jar with a tight-fitting lid.

Put the loosely packed Echinacea leaf and finely chopped root into the jar. Fill with 80 proof vodka or rum and tightly fasten the lid. Keep the herb covered and shake the jar daily for 2 months. Add more alcohol when needed to keep the jar full. Strain the herbs. Keep the extract covered in a cool, dark place.

Elecampane, *Inula helenium*

Elecampane, a member of the sunflower family Asteraceae, is also commonly known as horse-heal, horse-elder, wild sunflower, starwort and elfdock. According to legend, the plant sprung up where the tears fell from Helen of Troy. The plant was considered sacred to the Celts and was thought to be associated with the fairy folk.

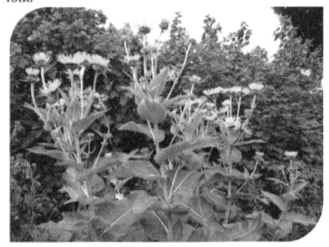

Elecampane is found in moist soil and shady places. It is cultivated in North America and is naturalized in the eastern United States growing in pastures, along roadsides, and at the base of eastern and southern facing slopes.

Identification: Elecampane is an upright herb that grows up to 6 feet (2m) in height. The large rough leaves are toothed and can be egg-shaped, elliptical, or lance-shaped. Lower leaves have a stalk, while the upper ones grow directly on the stem. Each leaf is up to 12 to 20 inches long (15cm-30cm) and 5 inches (12cm) wide. The upper side of the leaf is hairy and green, while the underside is whitish and velvety.

Flower heads are up to 3 inches (7 cm) in diameter and contain 50 to 100 yellow ray flowers and 100 to 250 yellow disc flowers. Elecampane blooms from June to August. The flowers are large, bright yellow, and resemble a double sunflower. The brown aromatic root branches below ground. It is large, thick, mucilaginous, and bitter with a camphoraceous odor and a floral background scent.

Edible Use: The root has been used in the making of absinthe and as a condiment. It stimulates pungent and bitter tastes, but it also has a sweet flavor due to its high polysaccharide content (inulin). Inulin, not to be confused with insulin, is a prebiotic that is used to feed and support healthy gut bacteria.

Medicinal Use: The elecampane root is the part most often used medicinally. Asian traditions also use the flowers, but I have had best results with the roots.

Elecampane root is useful fresh and dried. It can be infused into honey, extracted in alcohol, made into cough syrup, or made into a tea.

In most cases, it is best to start with a small dose and slowly increase it until the best results are obtained without nausea or overly drying effects.

Elecampane contains alantolactone and isoalantolactone, which is antibacterial, antifungal, and acts as a vermifuge (against parasites). These compounds also demonstrate anti-cancer activity, helping with apoptosis (programmed cell death).

Asthma, Bronchitis, Mucus, Whooping Cough, Influenza, and Tuberculosis: Elecampane root is useful as an expectorant and cough preventative in asthma, bronchitis, whooping cough, and tuberculosis. It lessens the need to cough by loosening phlegm and making the cough productive. It is beneficial for any respiratory illness 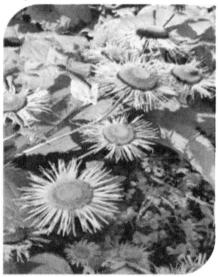 with excess mucus discharge. Not recommended for dry coughs. It soothes bronchial tube linings, reduces swelling and irritation of the respiratory tract, cleanses the lungs, and fights harmful organisms in the respiratory tract. For acute coughs, use small, frequent doses. It is also useful to support lung health in asthma patients (as is mullein).

Stimulates Digestion and Appetite: While elecampane is mostly valued for its effects on the respiratory system, it is also valuable for treating digestive system problems. It is warming, draining, and bitter.

Use elecampane for poor digestion, poor absorption, poor appetite, mucus in the digestive system, excess gas, and lethargy or sluggishness of the digestive system.

Elecampane strengthens digestion and improves absorption which is beneficial in malnourished or undernourished patients. It also treats nausea and diarrhea.

Type 2 Diabetes: The high inulin content in elecampane is helpful for patients with high blood sugar and for type 2 diabetes patients. Inulin slows down sugar metabolism, reduces blood glucose spikes and decreases insulin resistance. It may also reduce inflammation associated with diabetes.

Intestinal Parasites: Elecampane is a vermifuge that eliminates intestinal parasites from the body, including hookworm, roundworm, threadworm, and whipworm.

Cancer: Elecampane contains alantolactone and isoalantolactone, which have been shown to help with programmed cell death (apoptosis) for certain cancers.

Harvesting: Harvest fresh elecampane root in the fall after the plant has produced seed, or in the early spring before leaves appear. I prefer roots that are two to three years old. Older roots are too woody, and younger roots lack their full medicinal potential. It is best to dig up some of the larger horizontal roots and leave the remaining roots so the plant can continue growing.

Warning: Large doses of elecampane can cause nausea, vomiting, and diarrhea.

Avoid use of elecampane during pregnancy since it can cause contractions and is a uterine stimulant.

Skin rashes have been reported in sensitive people. Persons with known allergies to plants in the Aster family should avoid using elecampane.

Elecampane can lower blood sugar and could interfere with blood sugar control in diabetics.

There are indications that elecampane may interfere with blood pressure control in some patients. Monitor blood pressure carefully while using elecampane.

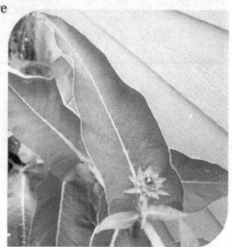

Do not use elecampane within 2 weeks before or after a scheduled surgery.

It may cause drowsiness – no not use with sedatives.

Evening Primrose, *Oenothera biennis*

Evening primrose is also known as evening star and sun drop. Evening primrose gets its name because its flowers usually open at dusk, after the sun is no longer on them. It grows in eastern and central North America and has naturalized to Europe. It is in the Onagraceae (Evening Primrose) Family.

Identification: *Oenothera biennis* is a biennial plant. In its first year, the leaves can grow up to 10 inches (25 cm) long. Leaves are lance-shaped, toothed, and form a rosette. In its second year, the flower stem has alternate, spirally-arranged leaves on a hairy, rough flower stem that is often tinged with purple.

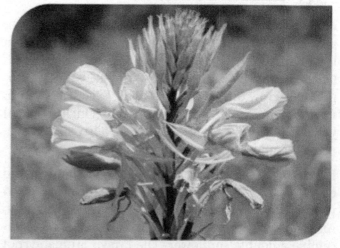

The leaves are reminiscent of willow leaves. This erect flower stem sometimes branches near the top of the plant and grows from 3 to 6 feet (0.9m to 1.8m) tall. It flowers from June to October.

The bright yellow flowers are partially to fully closed during the heat of the day. Flowers have four petals and are 1 to 2 inches (2.5 cm to 5 cm) across. They grow in a many-flowered terminal panicle. The fragrant flowers last only 1 to 2 days. Seedpods are long and narrow.

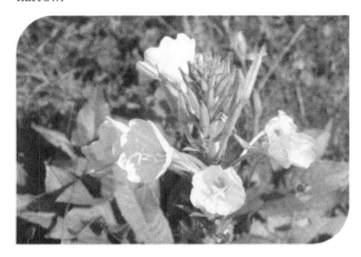

Edible Use: All parts of evening primrose are edible, including the flowers, leaves, stalks, oil, root, and seedpods. Roots can be eaten either cooked or boiled. Its flowers and flower buds are good raw in salads. Young seedpods can be cooked or steamed. Second year stems can be peeled and eaten fresh. Its seeds are edible and oily. Leaves aren't usually eaten due to their texture but they can be if boiled a few times.

Medicinal Use: Evening primrose oil comes from the seeds of the evening primrose, which contain gamma linolenic acid (GLA) - an omega 6 fatty acid also found in borage. Flowers, roots, bark, and leaves are also used medicinally.

Balancing Women's Hormones, PCOS, PMS, and Menopause: Evening primrose oil helps balance hormones in women. It naturally treats symptoms of PMS, including breast tenderness, water retention and bloating, acne, irritability, depression, moodiness, and headaches.

It is also useful in the treatment of polycystic ovarian syndrome (PCOS), helping with fertility and in normalizing the menstrual cycle. It helps ease the symptoms of menopause as well, like hot flashes, moodiness, and sleep disturbance.

Hair Loss in Men and Women: Evening primrose attacks the hormonal causes of male pattern baldness and androgenetic alopecia in women. By balancing the hormones, it prevents further hair loss and, in some people, helps hair grow back. It is best used both internally and externally (rub on the scalp daily along with diluted rosemary essential oil).

Skin Diseases, Eczema, Psoriasis, Acne: Evening primrose oil works well for people with skin problems such as acne, eczema, dermatitis, and psoriasis. It balances the hormonal causes of these diseases, reduces inflammation, and promotes healing while reducing symptoms such as itching, redness, and swelling.

Arthritis and Osteoporosis: Evening primrose oil is a good supplement for people with rheumatoid arthritis and osteoporosis. It is anti-inflammatory and reduces pain and stiffness. It also balances the hormones that cause bone loss in osteoporosis. It also seems to help with calcium absorption and is best combined with fish oil.

Gastro-Intestinal Disorders: The bark and leaves are astringent and healing. They are effective in treating gastro-intestinal disorders caused by muscle spasms of the stomach or intestines. They calm the spasms and allow better digestion.

Whooping Cough: Evening primrose is an expectorant. A syrup made from the flowers helps treat whooping cough symptoms and is easier than a tincture or tea to get young children to swallow. Boil the flowers in a small amount of water, strain, and sweeten with raw honey.

Asthma and Allergies: Use leaf and bark tea to treat asthma. The tea relieves bronchial spasms and opens the airways. It does not cure the asthma, only treats the symptoms. It seems to work best for asthma with allergic causes.

Blood Pressure and Cholesterol: Regular consumption of evening primrose oil helps reduce blood cholesterol levels and lowers blood pressure.

Best results are achieved by long-term use; it is not intended for acute situations.

Diabetic Neuropathy: Evening primrose oil helps treat nerve pain specifically due to diabetes.

Harvesting, Preparation, and Storage: The seeds of evening primrose ripen from August to October. Collect them when ripe and press for oil before they dry out. Flowers must be picked in full bloom.

Gather the leaves and stem "bark" when the flowering stems have grown up. Strip the "bark" of evening primrose and dry for later use; the leaves are also harvested and dried at that time. Dig the roots in the second year when they are larger and more potent.

Recipes. How to Make Cold-Pressed Evening Primrose Seed Oil: Grind fresh seeds. You can use a flourmill, sausage grinder, auger type juicer, coffee grinder, or blender to grind the seeds into a paste. It may take several passes through the grinder to get a fine grind. Add a tiny amount of water only if necessary, to facilitate grinding. Roll the ground seeds into a ball and knead them by hand to release the oil, catching it in a small bowl. Knead and squeeze the seeds until the oil is released, this may take some time. Place the seed paste into a seed bag or use a coffee filter and tighten it to release even more oil into the bowl. When you have gathered as much oil as possible, filter it through a fresh filter to remove any remaining seed remnants. The standard dosage for internal use is 1 gram of oil daily, broken into 2 to 3 doses.

Strong Evening Primrose Tea. (1-ounce bark and leaves, crushed or chopped into small pieces, 1-pint (500 ml) of water). Bring the water and herbs to a boil and reduce the heat to a low simmer. Simmer the herbs for 10 minutes. Allow the tea to cool and strain out the herbs. Keep the tea refrigerated until needed and use within three days.

Fennel,
Foeniculum vulgare

Fennel is a commonly used vegetable in the Apiaceae /Umbelliferae (Celery/Carrot/Parsley) Family. It has a licorice flavor and is very fragrant. It is found across the United States and Canada. I grow it in my garden, but am also able to find it along roadsides, riverbanks, and pasture lands.

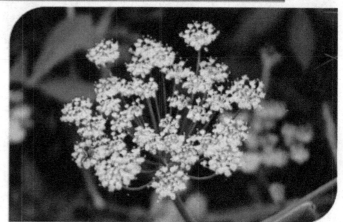

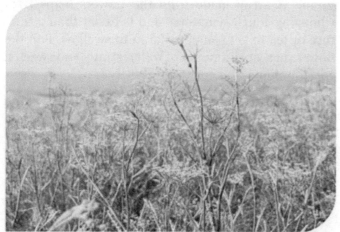

Identification: Fennel is a flowering perennial herb with yellow flowers. It looks a lot like dill, except for the bulb. The leaves are feathery, and finer than dill leaves. The stems are erect, smooth and green and grow to a height of eight feet (2.4m).

The leaves are finely dissected with threadlike segments. Most, but not all varieties form a stem-bulb that sits on the ground or is lifted by a segment of stem. Leaf branches fan out from the stem, forming the bulb. Flowers appear on umbels, 2 to 6 inches (5 cm to 15 cm) in diameter. The umbels are terminal and compound, with each section containing 20 to 50 tiny yellow flowers. The fruit is a small seed, approximately 1/5 to 1/3 inch-long (0.6 cm to 0.9 cm) with grooves along its length.

Edible Use: The stems, leaves, and seeds are edible. I prefer to roast the bulbs and use the seeds for seasoning.

Medicinal Use: The seeds and root are used to prepare remedies, but eating the plant is also healthy.

Digestive Problems: An infusion made from the seeds is effective in the treatment of digestive problems. Take it after meals for the treatment of indigestion, heartburn, and flatulence.

It is also effective for constipation and stomach pains. In addition to using the infusion, if you have digestive problems add fennel seeds to your cooking.

Nursing Mothers and Colic: For the treatment of colic, have the mother drink Fennel Infusion. It not only relieves the baby's colic, but it also increases the milk flow. Non-nursing babies can take a spoonful of the infusion to relieve the symptoms.

Sore Throats, Laryngitis, Gum Problems: I also use Fennel Infusion as a treatment for sore throats. Gargle with the infusion to treat the infection and pain. This treatment is also effective for sore gums.

Urinary Tract Problems, Kidney Stones: For urinary tract infections, kidney stones, and other urinary tract problems, use a decoction of the fennel root.

Menstrual Problems and Premenstrual Tension: Fennel has the ability to regulate the menstrual cycle and the hormones affecting it. I prescribe Fennel Seed Tea for a variety of menstrual problems including cramping, PMS, pain fluid retention and other menstrual symptoms. Fennel contains estrogen-like chemicals that work to restore the hormonal balance

Detoxifying, Diuretic: Fennel is a strong diuretic and detoxifier. It cleans toxins from the body and flushes them out through the urinary tract. Drink Fennel Seed Tea up to three times daily to detoxify the body and remove excess fluids.

Eyesight, Eyewash, Conjunctivitis, Eye Inflammations: To strengthen eyesight, eat fennel with your meals.

For inflammations and eye infections, use Fennel Seed Tea as an eyewash. It treats conjunctivitis, infections and reduces inflammations of the eye.

Harvesting: Harvest fennel seeds in autumn when they are fully mature. Dry them and store in an air-tight container in a cool, dark place.

Warning: Rarely people have had problems with photo-dermatitis while taking fennel seed. Fennel has hormonal effects and should not be consumed by pregnant women.

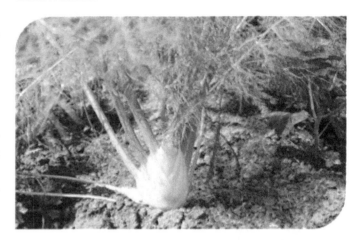

Recipes. Fennel Infusion: You need 1 teaspoon crushed fennel seeds and 1 cup boiling water. Pour the boiling water over the fennel seeds and allow the infusion to steep, covered, for 10 to 15 minutes. Drink 3 cups daily. Take after meals for digestive issues.

Fennel Root Decoction: To make the decoction get 2 ounces (56g) chopped fennel root, fresh and 1-quart (1 Liter) water. Bring the fennel root and water to a boil and turn the heat down to a simmer. Simmer the decoction for 1 hour. Turn off the heat and strain out the root. Store the decoction in the refrigerator for up to 1 week.

Feverfew,
Tanacetum parthenium

Feverfew is an herb that is widely used for migraines. It grows along roadsides, in rocky and disturbed soil, and is cultivated in some home herb and ornamental gardens. Also known as Chrysanthemum parthenium, wild chamomile, and bachelor's buttons. It is a member of the Aster/Daisy Family.

Identification: Feverfew grows into a bushy shape approximately 1 to 3 feet (0.3m to 0.9m) tall. It has round, leafy stems that grow from a taproot. The leaves

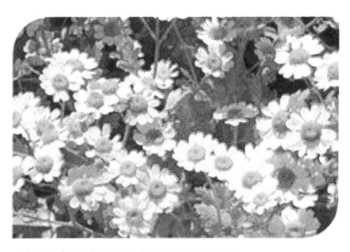

Flower of Feverfew 1Feverfew by Vision, CC 2.5

are yellow-green and pinnately divided into slightly rounded divisions. The upper leaves are more lobed and toothed than lower leaves. Leaves have a distinctive bitter aroma and taste. Flowers bloom in summer.

The flowers look like small daisies with a large yellow disk and short white rays. The center disk is flat, unlike chamomiles, which have conical central disks.

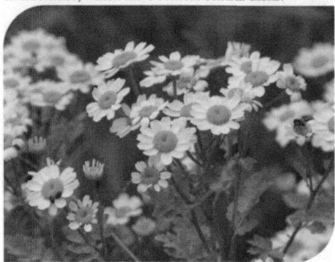

Edible Use: Feverfew leaves are edible but are very bitter.

Medicinal Use: The leaves and flowers are used medicinally. Typical doses are 2 to 3 leaves per day, with a proportionally reduced dose for children over the age of three.

Migraines and Tension Headaches: Taking feverfew regularly works well as a preventative for migraine headaches, as does butterbur. It must be taken regularly to work.

Feverfew may work in a few ways: as an anti-inflammatory, by inhibiting smooth muscle contraction, as an analgesic, and by inhibiting blood platelet aggregation. It may also help via other mechanisms still being studied.

Use the flowers and leaves fresh or dried. To prevent migraines, chew 1 to 4 leaves per day, or drink 1 cup of Feverfew Leaf Tea daily, or use a daily tincture.

For people with migraines simply keep dried leaves or a feverfew tincture on hand with you.

If mouth sores develop from chewing leaves regularly, switch to a powdered or tinctured form. The tea, leaf,

or tincture may also be used as a treatment for tension headaches.

Fevers, Cold and Flu Pain (and Colic): Feverfew gets its name from its traditional use treating fevers. Hot Feverfew Tea helps break a fever and treats the aches and pains associated with cold and flu. It is anti-inflammatory and analgesic. For colic in babies and young children, try just a few drops of a cold infusion.

Menstrual Cramps and to Regulate the Menses: Feverfew is both a uterine stimulant and a pain reliever and is particularly good at relieving painful menstrual cramping and in bringing on menses.

Feverfew shouldn't be used if you are pregnant, as it can stimulate uterine contraction and directly affect the baby.

Harvesting: Harvest feverfew leaves and flowers shortly after the flowers appear in early summer. Dry a supply for future use. You can also powder the dried leaves and encapsulate them.

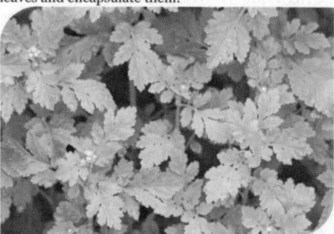

Warning: Some people have an allergic reaction to feverfew and dermatitis can also occur with skin contact. Chewing the leaves can cause mouth sores in some people. If you are allergic to ragweed, marigold, or chrysanthemum, you may also react to feverfew.

Do not use during pregnancy as it causes contractions. Do not use on people who have blood coagulation problems.

Recipes. Feverfew Tea: Steep 1 heaping teaspoon of feverfew leaves and flowerheads in 1 cup of hot water. Allow the infusion to cool to lukewarm, then drink it or apply as directed.

Garlic, *Allium sativum*

Garlic has strong medicinal value, and it tastes great. Most people would benefit greatly by eating more garlic, no matter how good or bad their health. I use garlic for nearly everything.

Most of the garlic that I use now is cultivated. It is found in nearly every herb garden and kitchen garden across the country and is easily found at supermarkets. Don't fall for prepared garlic, however. Chop it fresh and make your own garlic products for maximum health.

Identification: The garlic plant grows to about 2 feet (0.6 meters) tall. It is a bulbous herb with four to twelve long, flat, sword-shaped leaves growing from an underground stem. The bulbs are rounded and contain approximately 15 smaller cloves. Each clove and the bulb is covered by a thin white or pinkish papery coat. Flowers appear in a cluster at the top of a 10-inch (25 cm) flower stalk. Flower stalks grow from a common point on each plant. The flowers are green-white or pinkish with six sepals and petals. Propagation is primarily by bulbs. Seeds are rarely produced.

Edible Use: The bulbs are the only part of the garlic eaten and are usually used for seasoning or as a condiment.

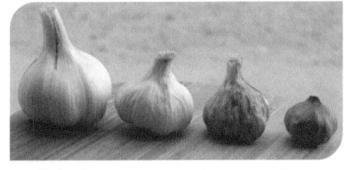

Medicinal Use: For internal use, I usually recommend that people simply eat more garlic in their foods. For best results, garlic should be chopped fine and allowed to rest for 10 minutes or so before cooking. Eating it raw is even better.

Chopping, and allowing time for the sulfurous compounds to develop in the garlic, will make it more potent. Some people complain of a strong garlic smell in the sweat when consuming garlic. This is a natural response and indicates that the body is using the beneficial components. To alleviate this complaint, eat fresh parsley with the garlic.

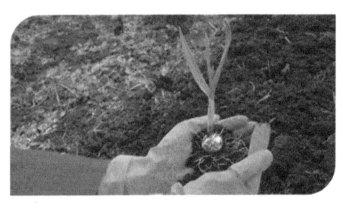

Taking Garlic as Medicine: In general, use garlic in any way that best suits you. People who don't like the strong flavor can put it into capsules, but I like using it fresh and chopped fine or crushed to release the beneficial sulfurous compounds.

You can also take it as a tincture. For people who like garlic, try chewing one whole raw clove at each meal or drinking garlic juice daily.

Treating Viral, Bacterial, and Parasitic Infections: Garlic is a potent antibiotic, antifungal, and anti-parasitic plant. Use garlic to treat infections of all kinds, including colds, flu, sore throats, bronchitis, stomach flu, and intestinal worms.

Thrush, Yeast, and Fungal Infections: Use garlic preparations topically to treat thrush infections and other types of yeast or fungal infections. Spread a paste of garlic on the affected area several times a day and eat garlic regularly to clear the infection internally.

Digestive Problems: Garlic improves digestion and is useful to relieve excessive gas, bloating, and other digestive upsets.

Lowers Blood Sugars in Diabetics: Garlic helps lower blood sugar in diabetics by improving the function of the pancreas and increasing the secretion of insulin.

This helps the body regulate blood sugar levels and alleviates the problems associated with high blood sugar. To be effective, garlic needs to be eaten at every meal in significant quantities. Adding a couple of cloves of pickled garlic to the meal is usually enough to get the full benefits.

Bronchitis, Whooping Cough, Congestion of All Causes: Garlic has a strong decongestant effect and expectorant action. It is useful for maladies where phlegm or mucous is a problem. Garlic also reduces fevers and kills off the underlying infection. It is also useful for bronchial asthma where the breathing passages have swollen making breathing difficult.

Elevated Blood Cholesterol Levels and Blood Pressure: Garlic effectively lowers blood cholesterol levels and blood pressure when consumed regularly.

Corns, Warts, and Acne: For corns, warts, and acne, rub a paste made from fresh mashed garlic on the affected spot. Garlic actually softens and soothes the skin and kills the viral or bacterial infection causing the problem.

Recipes: Garlic Infusion. Chop or grind garlic cloves and allow them to rest for 10 to 15 minutes before continuing. Place the garlic into a pot and cover with water. Heat the water gently to a simmer, then turn off the heat. Allow the garlic and water to steep overnight. Use 2 to 4 ml of this infusion, 3 times a day with meals. Keep the Infusion in the refrigerator for up to three days or in the freezer for up to a month.

Garlic Tincture: Chop 1 cup of garlic cloves fine and allow to rest for 10 to 15 minutes. Place the garlic cloves in a pint (500ml) jar with a tight-fitting lid. Cover the chopped garlic with apple cider vinegar, preferably with the mother (live vinegar). Allow the jar to steep for 4 to 6 weeks, shaking it several times a week. Take 1 tablespoon of garlic tincture with each meal.

Goldenrod, *Solidago* spp.

Goldenrods comprise about 100 species or more that grow throughout North America in open areas like meadows, prairies, and savannas. I primarily use *Solidago canadensis*, which is the most common goldenrod in North America. It is in the Aster/Daisy Family and is also known as goldruthe, woundwort, and solidago. Goldenrods take the blame for a lot of allergies, but most of it is undeserved. There are people allergic to goldenrod and they should not use the plant. However, most of the allergies are caused by ragweed and other similar flowering plants. Goldenrod are pollinated by bees and do not release pollen into the air like the ragweeds. Furthermore, Goldenrod can be used against allergies caused by ragweed.

Identification: I often find goldenrod in open areas and along trailsides. I identify it by its unique aroma, taste, and its visual properties – like its height and its large sprays of yellow flower clusters. Crushing a goldenrod leaf releases a salty, balsam-like fragrance.

Any goldenrod species can be used medicinally; however, it is necessary to differentiate the plant from similar toxic plants, including ragwort and groundsel. If you are unsure of your identification, use a local field guide. Goldenrod plants have alternate, simple leaves that are usually toothed. They can also be smooth or hairy.

The leaves at the base of the plant are longer, shortening as they climb the plant, with no leaf stem and 3 distinct parallel veins. The shape can vary from species to species. The stems are unbranched, until the plant flowers. Flower heads are composed of yellow ray florets arranged around disc florets. Each flower head may contain a few florets per head or up to 30, depending on the species. The flower head is usually 1/2 inch (1.25 cm) or less in diameter, although some varieties are larger. The inflorescence is usually a raceme or a panicle. Plant size varies by species, usually growing 2 to 5 feet (0.6 meters to 1.5meters) tall. Some varieties spread aggressively by runners, while others grow in clumps that expand outward each year.

Toxic Look-Alikes: Goldenrod has many look-alikes and some of them are deadly. Groundsel, life root, staggerweed, and ragwort are regional names for deadly look-alike plants in the Senecio genus. Ragwort and groundsels usually have fewer and smaller flower heads and bloom earlier in the season.

These are not hard rules, however, so it can be difficult to identify the plants and distinguish them from other local varieties. You should be very sure of your plant identification before harvesting.

Edible Use: Goldenrod flowers are edible and can be eaten lightly fried or in a salad. It is also used as a flavoring for alcoholic beverages such as cordials and mead, and in fermented homemade soda. Leaves can be cooked and eaten like spinach.

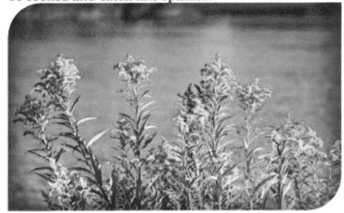

Medicinal Use: I use the leaves and flowers in my medicinal preparations; however, the roots are also used. I use goldenrod to made medicinal tea and tinctures. For children, it can be infused into raw honey or made into a syrup.

Urinary Tract and Kidneys: Goldenrod has astringent and antiseptic properties, that are useful in treating urinary tract infections and bladder infections. It is also effective in restoring balance to the kidneys and in prevention of kidney stones. It is a good choice for chronic conditions and long-term use, though care should be taken as it is a diuretic. Other treatments might be more useful for acute UTI and kidney infections.

Skin, Wounds, and Stopping Bleeding: Goldenrod is an herb of choice to treat and help heal skin wounds, burns, open sores, cuts, boils and other skin irritations. The herb acts as an anti-inflammatory, antibacterial, and antifungal. It helps wounds heal quickly and soothes the irritation. I use goldenrod decoction as a wash, make a poultice, or sometimes use the powdered dried leaves directly on skin wounds. Its common name of "woundwort" came from its ability to stop bleeding when applied to a wound (its dried, powdered form works best as a styptic). You can also use goldenrod to make an ointment or salve. Roots were traditionally used for burns.

Colds, Allergies, and Bronchial Congestion: Goldenrod Tincture is a good choice for treating the symptoms of seasonal allergies and colds. It calms runny eyes and noses, and the sneezes that are triggered by summer and fall allergies.

It is an antiseptic and an expectorant and contains quercetin and rutin, which are natural antihistamines. It also treats sore throats. Goldenrod can also be taken as a tea when needed. For treating a sore throat, try combining it with sage.

Once cooled a bit, the tea can be used as a gargle for laryngitis and pharyngitis (sore throats). Goldenrod helps the body get rid of respiratory congestion caused by allergies, sinus infections, colds and the flu. It works much like Yerba Santa to dry bronchial and respiratory secretions and to expel existing mucous.

Diarrhea: Goldenrod stimulates the digestive systems while calming internal inflammation and irritation that causes diarrhea. It is anti-inflammatory and anti-microbial, so it attacks the symptoms and causes.

Boosts the Cardiovascular System: Goldenrod is a good source of rutin, a powerful antioxidant that improves the cardiovascular and cerebrovascular system. It supports circulation and increases capillary strength. Peoples with this need drink Goldenrod Tea daily, as long as they do not have problems with blood pressure.

Yeast Infections and Anti-Fungal: Goldenrod's antifungal properties make it effective against yeast infections such as *Candida*. Drink the tea or take the decoction daily and use powdered goldenrod, as needed, for external infections. A gargle can be used for oral thrush (Usnea also works well for thrush).

Joint Pain: This herb is anti-inflammatory, and works well to reduce pain and swelling, especially in the joints. It is useful to treat gout, arthritis, and other

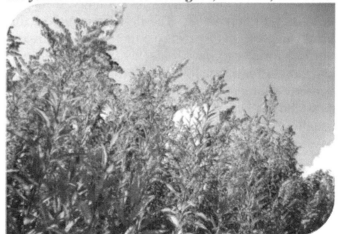

joint pains. Take internally and topically apply a poultice or wash directly to the affected joints.

Harvesting: Harvest healthy leaves and flowers that are free of powdery mildew or other diseases. Pick the leaves throughout the spring and summer and harvest flowers in the late summer or early autumn, just as the flowers open. Leave some flowers on the plant to produce seeds and guarantee a crop the next year. Roots are harvested in early spring or autumn. Hang the plants to dry or use a dehydrator on the lowest setting to dry them for long-term storage.

Warning: Goldenrod is a diuretic and can be overly drying when used long-term as a daily beverage or tea. Do not use goldenrod during pregnancy or when nursing. Consult your doctor if you have a chronic kidney disorder. Do not use goldenrod if you are allergic to any members of the Asteraceae family.

Be sure of your plant identification. There are poisonous look-alikes. Goldenrod can increase blood pressure in some people.

Recipes. Goldenrod Tea: You will need 2 cups of boiling water and 1 Tablespoon of fresh goldenrod or 2 teaspoons of dried goldenrod. Bring the water to a boil and pour over the goldenrod. Allow the herbs to infuse for 15 minutes. Strain and serve. Use up to three times a day. This tea is slightly bitter. Adding an equal amount of mint to the herbs improves the flavor.

Goldenrod Decoction: Ingredients: 1-ounce goldenrod herb (leaves or flowers), 1-pint (500ml) of water. Place the herbs in a non-reactive pot with the water over medium heat. Bring the mixture to a boil. Turn the temperature down to a low simmer for 20 minutes. Cool the decoction and strain out the herbs. Store in the refrigerator for up to 3 days. Use 1 to 2 teaspoons per dose, 3 times a day.

Greater Burdock, *Arctium lappa*

Arctium lappa belongs to Asteraceae (Daisy) Family. It is commonly known as greater burdock, edible burdock, lappa, beggar's buttons, thorny burr, or happy major. It is a Eurasian species and is cultivated in gardens for its root, which is used as a vegetable. This plant has become an invasive weed in many places in North America. It is a giant weed with much medicinal potential.

Identification: Greater burdock is a biennial plant. It is tall, and can reach 10 feet (3meters). Its stems are branched, rough and usually sparsely hairy. It flowers from July to September. The fleshy tap-root of this plant can grow up to 3 feet (0.9 meters) deep. Greater Burdock forms a 1.5-inch-wide (3.75 cm) single flower-like flat cluster of small purple flowers surrounded by a rosette of bracts. Leaves of greater burdock are alternate and stalked. They are triangular–broadly oval, usually cordate, and have undulating margins. They have a white-grey-cottony underside and first year growth is in rosettes.

The fruit is flattish, gently curved and is grey-brown in color. It has dark-spotted achene with short yellow hooked hairs on tip. Greater burdock is found almost everywhere, especially in areas soils that are usually rich in nitrogen. Its preferred habitat is in disturbed areas.

Edible Use: The leaves, stems, seeds, and roots are all edible. Young first-year roots and leaves are good raw in salads, but they become too fibrous as they mature and need to be cooked before eating.

The leaves and stalks are also good either raw or cooked. I prefer to remove the outer rind before cooking or eating. The sprouted seeds are also eaten.

Medicinal Use: Greater Burdock is antibacterial and antifungal, helps with digestion and gas, is a diuretic, and regulates blood sugar. It is a powerful

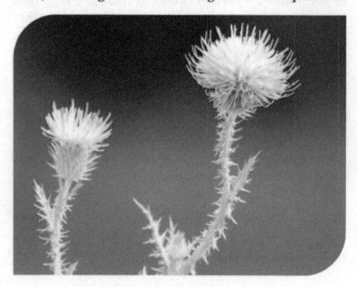

detoxifier. The dried root is most often used for medicine, but the leaves and fruit can also be used.

Detoxing and Liver Cleanser: Its root is particularly good at helping to eliminate heavy metals and other resilient toxins from the body.

It helps with conditions caused by an overload of toxins, such as sore throat and other infections, boils, rashes, and other skin problems.

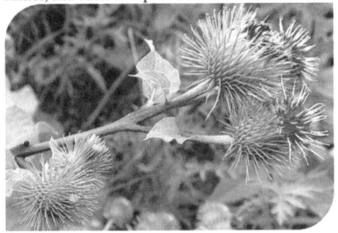

Burdock flowers, Pethan, GNUFL 1.2

Cancer Treatment: Greater burdock is known to kill cancer cells. It flushes away toxins from the body, increases blood circulation to normal cells, protects the organs, and improves the health of the whole body. It is used to treat breast cancers, colon cancer, and even the deadly pancreatic cancer with good results.

I feel confident that it would be effective against other cancers as well. In treating cancer, the greatest success seems to come when herbs are used in combination to kill the cancer cells and support the body.

Try using greater burdock in combination with sheep sorrel and slippery elm to kill the cancer and detox the body during treatment. Remember to also eat a highly nutritious diet with a high concentration of vegetables and fruits and limited meats and fats.

Turkey Tail and Reishi Mushrooms are other cancer go-tos for me. Dosage: Mix 1/4 cup of Anti-Cancer Decoction with 1/4 cup of distilled water. Drink 3 times a day: 2 hours before breakfast, 2 hours after lunch and before bedtime on an empty stomach. Wait at least 2 hours after taking the decoction before eating again.

Anemia: Greater burdock has a high concentration of bioavailable iron. People with iron deficiency anemia are able to increase their iron levels rapidly by taking daily supplements of greater burdock powder or eating greater burdock as a vegetable.

Skin Diseases: Greater burdock is a very soothing herb for the skin. It has mucilaginous properties that enhance its ability to cure skin diseases such as herpes, eczema, psoriasis, acne, impetigo, ringworm, boils, insect bites, burns, and bruises. Use greater burdock tea as a wash and take it internally to clear the body of the toxins that are causing the skin problems. For bruises, burns, and sores, crush the seeds and use as a poultice on the affected skin.

Diabetes: Greater burdock root helps improve digestion and lower blood sugar in diabetics. For this use the fresh root is best, but 1 to 2 grams of dried powdered root can also be taken 3 times daily.

Strengthens the Immune System and Protects the Organs: This herb strengthens the immune system and the lymphatic system, which helps rid the body of toxins and ward off diseases. It also cleans the blood. It cleand and protects the spleen and helps it remove dangerous pathogens from the body. It improves blood quality, liver health, blood circulation, and fights inflammation.

Stimulates the Kidneys, Relieves Fluid Retention: Greater burdock stimulates the kidneys, helping get rid of excess fluids in the body. This reduces swellings, increases urine output, and flushes waste and toxins from the body.

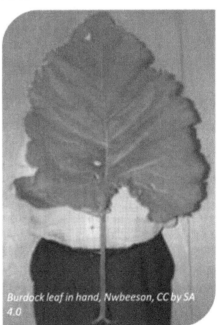

Burdock leaf in hand, Nwbeeson, CC by SA 4.0

Greater Burdock Tea is a natural diuretic.

Osteoarthritis and Degenerative Joint Disease: The anti-inflammatory properties of greater burdock are powerful enough to reduce the inflammation of osteoarthritis. Patients show remarkable improvement when they consume three cups of Greater Burdock Root Tea daily.

Improvement is slow and steady, taking about two months to achieve maximum benefits.

Sore Throats and Tonsillitis: For acute tonsillitis and other sore throats, try Greater Burdock Tea. It relieves pain, inflammation, coughing, and speeds healing. The greater burdock also acts as an antibacterial to kill the harmful bacteria and cure the infection.

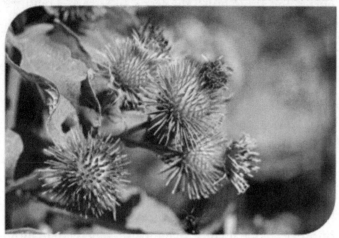

Harvesting: The root must be harvested before it withers at the end of the first year. The best time is after it seeds until late autumn when the roots become very fibrous. Immature flower stalks are harvested in late spring before the flowers appear. Care must be taken when harvesting the seeds. They have tiny,

hooked hairs that can latch onto the mucus membranes if inhaled.

Recipes. Anti-Cancer Decoction: To make 1-gallon (4 liters) you need 1-ounce greater burdock root, powdered, 3/4 ounces (21g) sheep sorrel, powdered, 1/4 ounces (7g) slippery elm bark, powdered and 1-gallon (4 liters) distilled water. Equipment: 8-pint (4 Liters) canning jars and lids, sterile, large pot, capable of holding 1 gallon (4 liters) or more, with a tight-fitting lid and boiling water canner.

Bring the greater burdock, sheep sorrel, and slippery elm bark to a boil in 1 gallon (4 liters) of distilled water, tightly covered. Boil the herbs, tightly covered, for 10 minutes, then turn off the heat and stir the mixture.

Cover tightly and let the decoction steep for 12 hours, stirring again after 6 hours. After 12 hours, bring it back to a boil and pour it through a fine mesh strainer or a coffee filter. Pour the decoction into pint (500ml) jars while still hot, leaving ½ inch (1.25 cm) headroom. Cap the jars. Process the jars in a boiling water bath for 10 minutes.

The decoction will keep for 1 year in sealed jars. Store in the refrigerator after opening. Dosage: Mix 1/4 cup of the decoction with 1/4 cup of distilled water. Drink 3 times a day: 2 hours before breakfast, 2 hours after lunch and before bedtime on an empty stomach. Wait at least 2 hours after taking the decoction before eating again.

Henbane,
Hyoscyamus niger

Henbane is poisonous, so it is advised that you use it with caution. Although native to Europe, it has been cultivated in North America for many years. It's a beautiful plant with a foul smell, and a member of the Solanaceae (Nightshade) family.

Identification: *Hyoscyamus niger* grows from 1 to 3 feet (0.9 meters) tall. A mature henbane plant has leafy, thick, hairy, widely-branched, erect stems. It is an annual and biannual and the biannual growth is used for medicine. Its foul-smelling lobed alternate leaves are grayish-green or yellowish-green in color and have white veins. They spread out like a rosette and are coarsely toothed, large, and wide, growing up

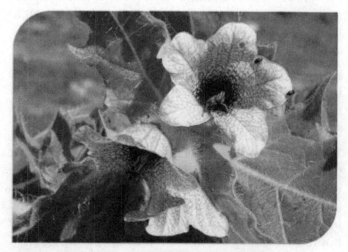

Henbane, photo by K.B. Simoglou - Own work, CC BY-SA 4.0,

to 6 inches (15 cm) wide and 8 inches (20 cm) long. The 5-petaled flowers are a funnel shape and are brownish-yellow in color with dark purple veins. Flowers have a long-spiked inflorescence arrangement in upper leaves with young flowers at the pointed end. Flowers are up to 2 inches (5 cm) across. It flowers from June thru September. The 5-lobed, urn-shaped fruit is 1 inch (2.5 cm). Each fruit is packed with hundreds of tiny black seeds. The roots of henbane are whitish in color. The main taproot is stout and branched. Henbane does not tolerate waterlogged soils. It likes pastures along fencerows and roadsides.

Medicinal Use: Because the plant is poisonous, it is important that all medicines be made precisely and the strength carefully regulated. I prefer to use this plant externally, where there is no danger.

The plant has strong pain-relieving qualities, and is used externally for muscle pains caused by strain or sprain. It has some good applications internally, but I do not recommend using it internally without the close supervision of a medical professional. The above ground parts are used for medicine.

Internal Use: The plant is used to relieve irritable bladders and the pain of cystitis. It is a mild diuretic, hypnotic, and anti-spasmodic. The hypnotic action is the same as belladonna, but with milder effects. Use with great care or find an alternative! Use can be fatal.

Gout, Neuralgia, and Arthritis Pains: External pain from gout, neuralgia, and arthritis are

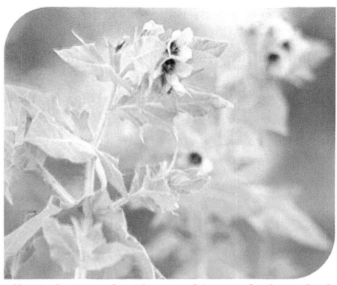

effectively treated with a poultice made from fresh henbane leaves. Crush the leaves and place them directly over the painful area.

Hemorrhoids: Try a poultice of crushed henbane leaves to reduce the swelling and pain of external hemorrhoids.

Harvesting: Collect the leaves, stems and flowers from the biennial plants when in full flower at the start of summer.

Warning: Henbane is poisonous. Use with great care and do not use internally.

Holy Basil, *Ocimum tenuiflorum / Ocimum sanctum*

Holy Basil, also known as Tulsi, is a variety of basil in the Lamiaceae (Mint) family. It is a perennial plant often cultivated for religious and medicinal use. It is not the same variety as Thai holy basil or Thai basil.

Holy basil is different from the sweet basil used as a cooking herb. Sweet basil also has medicinal properties but is a different variety of the plant.

Identification: Holy basil grows erect in shrub form up to 1 to 2 feet (0.3m-0.6m). The ovate leaves are green or purple, petioled, and up to 2 inches (5cm) long. The margin is usually, but not always, toothed. The anise scented leaves are strongly aromatic and have a spicy, slightly bitter flavor. They grow in close whorls at the base of reddish or brownish-purple stems. Tiny purple flowers grow on an elongated raceme above the leaves. The flower stems are red and hairy.

Edible Use: Holy basil is edible and can be used as an herb, however its flavor is more bitter than other basils. It is often chewed or used in herbal teas. The dried and ground leaves can be used as a flavoring and stored for later use.

Medicinal Use: Holy basil has many medicinal uses, both internally and externally. It is loaded with vitamins and antioxidants. In addition to treating many diseases, it can prevent disease through its immune system benefits.

Holy basil can be taken as a tea, eaten as a vegetable or flavoring, or taken as a supplement. Dried and crushed holy basil is often placed in capsules for daily supplement use. For preventative use, take 300 to 2,000 mg of dried holy basil daily. For treatment use, take 600 to 1,800 mg two to three times daily.

Inflammation: Holy basil is a powerful anti-inflammatory when taken internally or when rubbed on the skin for swellings and inflammation. Used regularly it leaves the skin soft and treats skin irritations and acne.

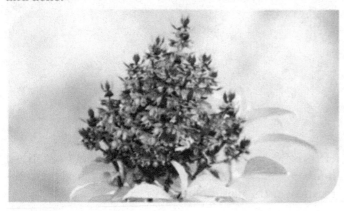

Skin Rashes, Ringworm: Rubbed against the skin, holy basil relieves irritations, soothes rashes, and provides anti-bacterial, anti-fungal, and antibiotic properties. It treats ringworm, poison oak, and other skin conditions.

Holy basil can be brewed in water, then added to your bath water or used as a face wash. A poultice of mashed holy basil leaves, applied directly to infected wounds, is effective in relieving infections and healing wounds. Consuming holy basil as an herb or supplement helps prevent skin problems.

Infections: Essential oils and phytonutrients in holy basil have excellent antibiotic, anti-fungal, and anti-bacterial properties.

Respiratory Disorders: Bronchitis, Asthma: Holy basil relieves congestion in the lungs caused by chronic or acute bronchitis. Additionally, it helps open breathing passages and allows for easier breathing. These benefits to the respiratory system are increased by the presence of healing oils and vitamins in the holy basil essential oil. These healing benefits extend to all damage in the lungs, including damage caused by smoking, environmental factors, or illness.

Stress and Heart Disease: Holy basil contains vitamins and antioxidants that protect the heart from the harmful effects of free radicals. One of these antioxidants, eugenol, is beneficial in reducing blood cholesterol levels. It lowers damaging LDL-cholesterol and raises the beneficial HDL-cholesterol. Users report a reduction in total cholesterol in the circulatory system, kidney, and liver.

In addition, these vitamins and antioxidants reduce the oxidative stress in the body. Holy basil soothes the nerves, reduces inflammation, and lowers blood pressure.

Cancer: Holy basil has anticancer potential, according to recent studies. It inhibits the growth of cancers, including oral cancer, and aids in cell death of cancerous cells.

Type 2 Diabetes: Holy basil works to reduce blood sugar in patients with prediabetes or type 2 diabetes. It helps with weight gain, reduces excess insulin in the blood, decreases insulin resistance, and helps keep blood sugar levels stable over the long term.

Dental Use: Holy basil, used correctly, protects the teeth and kills the bacteria responsible for cavities, plaque, tartar, and bad breath. It also promotes healthy gums. Use holy basil for dental care in moderation. Avoid chewing the leaves and do not keep it in the mouth for long periods. Prolonged contact can damage the teeth.

Detoxifier, Diuretic, and Reduces Risk of Kidney Stones: As a detoxifier and mild diuretic, holy basil reduces the levels of uric acid in the body. Uric acid is mainly responsible for the growth of kidney stones. Other components of holy basil help dissolve the stones, while it also helps relieve the pain from kidney stones as they pass. Holy basil increases urination, flushing toxins from the body and cleansing the kidneys. It helps protect the health of the kidneys and the liver.

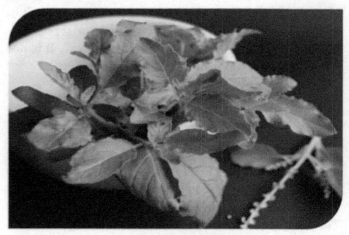

Pain Reliever: Holy basil has pain relieving properties that work well for headaches and minor pains. It helps relieve migraines, sinus headaches, and kidney pain.

Anti-Depressant Effects: Holy basil has known anti-depressant and anti-anxiety properties. It helps users feel less anxious and more relaxed in social situations. Holy basil also relieves stress from physical, mental, and emotional sources.

Eye Inflammations, Cataracts, Macular Degeneration, Glaucoma, Vision: Problems: Taken internally and regularly as a tea or as a supplement, holy basil helps prevent eye problems such as cataracts, macular degeneration, glaucoma, vision problems, and ophthalmia. Boils, conjunctivitis, and other eye inflammations or infections are treated by soaking holy basil in boiled water, then using the water to wash the eye. Holy basil contains high amounts of vitamins A and C, along with high antioxidant content and essential oils that are especially beneficial for the eyes.

Stomach and Digestive System: Holy basil is beneficial to the stomach and digestive system by naturally decreasing stomach acid and increasing mucus secretion. This naturally helps decrease number the effects of peptic ulcers. Eat the whole plant for relief from peptic ulcers, diarrhea, nausea, or vomiting.

Harvesting: Harvest holy basil from a source grown away from pollutants, pesticides, and herbicides. Look for vibrant green leaves without any holes or dark spots. Harvest the young leaves and stems from the top of the plant or cut the stems at ground level. Fresh

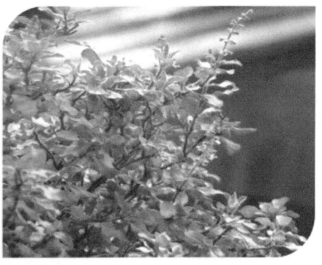

holy. Basil will keep for several days in the refrigerator or it can be dried for future use.

Recipes. Holy Basil Tea: 2 to 3 teaspoons of dried holy basil leaves, 1 cup boiling water. Pour boiling water over dried holy basil leaves and allow the mixture to steep for five to six minutes. Strain and enjoy.

Warning: Holy basil is considered safe for eating and medicinal uses. It should be avoided during pregnancy, when trying to become pregnant, or when breast-feeding because the effects on the child are unknown.

Holy basil can lower blood sugar levels and should be used with care when taking insulin or anti-diabetes drugs. People with hypothyroidism should not use holy basil. It may lower thyroxine levels and worsen the condition. Holy basil can interfere with blood clotting. Stop using holy basil at least 2 weeks before a scheduled surgery.

Hops, *Humulus lupulus*

Wild hops belong to the Cannabaceae (Hemp) Family. Hops are native to Europe, western Asia, and North America. Hops are a bine plant (versus a vine). They have a branching stem with stiff hairs that face downward and provide stability. These allow the plant to climb. Hops grow from 15 to 25 feet (4.5 meters to 7.6 meters) high.

Identification: Hops have green, opposite, lobed leaves. Leaves have 3 to 5 lobes with finely toothed edges and pointed tips. Male and female hops flowers are on separate plants. Male flowers grow in 3 to 5 inches (7.5 cm to 12.5 cm) panicles. The female flower (seed cone) resembles a small pine cone. Flowers are 1½ to 3 inches (3.75 to 7.5 cm) long with overlapping, yellowish-green bracts with a small fruit (achene) at the base. The flowers have a sweet smell.

Edible Use: The female flowers (seed cones or strobiles) are used for tea and for brewing beer. Young leaves and shoots are sometimes used cooked or eaten raw.

Extracts ad oils from hops are used as a flavoring in non-alcoholic beverages and sweets.

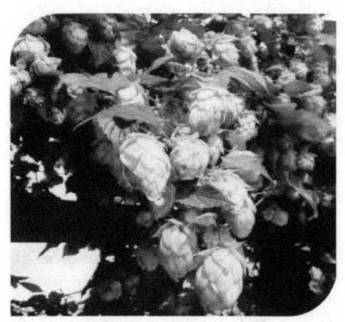

Hops, CCO Creative Commons, own work by moritz320

Bruises, Boils, and Inflammation: A poultice made of crushed hops helps heal bruises, boils, inflamed tissue, and arthritic joints.

Asthma, PMS, and Muscle Spasms: Hops are an antispasmodic and relieve menstrual cramping, muscle spasms, and bronchial spasms from asthma. It also has phytoestrogenic properties, similar to soy.

Harvesting: Time of harvest varies with the climate. Only the female seed cones are harvested and used in brewing, and both the pollinated and unpollinated hop flowers (strobili) are harvested.

Recipes: Valerian and Hops Infusion: 1-quart (1 Liter) of water, 1 heaping tablespoon of fresh hops, 1 heaping tablespoon of chopped valerian root, raw honey or maple syrup, if desired. Bring a quart (1 Liter) of water to a boil and add the herbs. Cover the pot and turn down the heat to a very low simmer. Simmer the infusion for 5 minutes, then turn the heat off.

Medicinal Use: Hops flowers are a sedative and stomachic, so they promote sleep and digestion. When used as a sedative, use fresh hops. For other medicinal uses, you may use dried hops.

Anxiety, Insomnia, and a Sedative: Fresh hops are a strong sedative. For insomnia and anxiety, try a combination of hops and valerian root at bedtime. Use dried hops for the anti-anxiety effects without the strong sedative effects.

Digestion: Hops are a very effective bitter. It is an excellent digestive.

IBS and Irritable Bladder: Hops treat the symptoms of Irritable Bowel Syndrome and irritable bladder. The bitter properties and the sedative qualities reduce spasms of both the bladder and the bowel, relieving the symptoms temporarily without affecting the underlying cause.

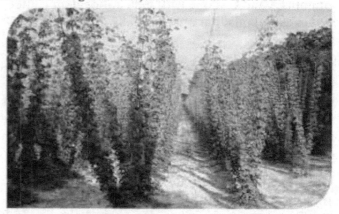

Hops field, Wikipedia Commons

Leave the pot covered and allow the herbs to steep for another 45 minutes. Sweeten the infusion with raw honey or pure maple syrup, if desired. Drink 1 to 1 ½ cups of the infusion at bedtime.

Horseradish, *Armoracia rusticana*

Horseradish is a perennial plant that belongs to Brassicaceae (Mustard) Family. It is a root vegetable that is used as a spice or condiment. It is native to the Southeastern Europe and Western Asia and has naturalized to North America. It is also known as Red Cole. My

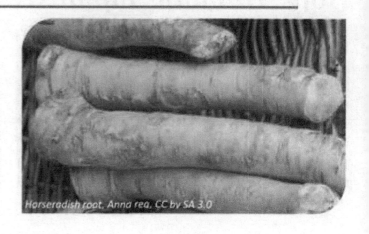

Horseradish root, Anna rea, CC by SA 3.0

favorite edible use for horseradish is as a condiment on meat. It is also one of the many ingredients which I use throughout the wintertime.

Identification: Horseradish is a perennial fast-growing plant that grows from 2 to 3 feet (0.6 m to 0.9 meters). Its flowering season is from May to June. It is self-fertile. The roots are thick and fleshy, a medium brown color on the outside, and smooth to corky on the outside. Roots are pure white on the inside and have a spicy flavor. The flowers of this plant are hermaphroditic (both male and female organs).

Edible Use: The root, leaves, and seeds are all edible, but the root is most often used.

Medicinal Use: The roots of this plant are antiseptic, digestive, diuretic, stimulant, laxative, rubefacient, and expectorant. It is a very powerful stimulant herb that controls bacterial infections, and it can be used both internally and externally.

Colds, Flu, Fevers, and Respiratory Infections: Horseradish infusion is of great value in the treatment of respiratory problems, colds, flu, and fevers. It is an expectorant, anti-bacterial, a weak diuretic, rids the body of excess mucus and fluids, and treats the underlying infection. It is also a key ingredient in my Fire Cider Recipe.

Urinary Tract Infections: The diuretic and anti-bacterial properties work well against urinary tract infections. Horseradish flushes the bacteria and toxins out of the body.

Arthritis, Pleurisy, Chilblains: For arthritis, chilblains, and pleurisy, apply a poultice made from freshly grated horseradish roots or rub the chest with Horseradish Massage Oil, when available.

The herb brings blood to the skin surface and increases blood circulation in the affected area. It warms the skin, decreases inflammation, and promotes healing.

Infected Wounds: The anti-microbial agents found in horseradish are beneficial in treating infected wounds. It acts as an antibiotic against bacteria and pathogenic fungi. Horseradish Vinegar works well for infected wounds.

Harvesting: Harvesting starts in November once the tops are frozen back. Harvesting can be continued through the winter when soils are not frozen. Before

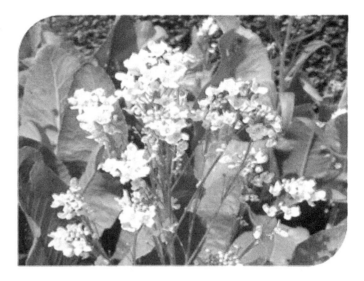

Horseradish plant, Pethan, CC by SA 3.0

digging, mow or cut the dried tops to the ground if still green. Roots are best harvested using a single-row potato digger. Freshly dug roots release valuable volatile oils and begin to lose potency. To avoid this, store them in a box of moist sand in a cool place. Keep the soil moist. Grate it fresh, as needed. Once grated, use it immediately.

Warning: People who have stomach ulcers or thyroid problems should not use this plant internally. Caution should be used when applying horseradish to the skin. It can cause skin irritation and blistering.

Fire Cider or Horseradish Vinegar – alter to your taste buds: Ingredients: ½ cup Grated Horseradish, ½ cup Grated Ginger, ¼ cup Minced Onions, ¼ cup Minced Garlic, 1 Chopped Lemon (rind on), 1 Tbs Black Peppercorns, ¼ tsp Cayenne Pepper and/or 2 Jalapeno Peppers (depends on your spice level), 1 Tbs Turmeric Powder, Raw honey to taste.

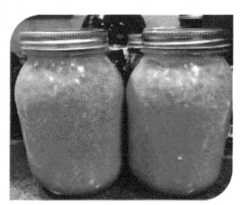

Put all of these into a large quart (liter) glass jar. Fill with organic raw apple cider vinegar. Let sit for 4 to 6 weeks, strain and store. Use within the year. I take it throughout the winter for wellness, usually about an ounce at a time.

Jerusalem Artichoke, *Helianthus tuberosus*

Also called sunroot, sunchoke, and earth apple, the Jerusalem artichoke is a species of sunflower found in Eastern North America. It is easy to cultivate in the garden. It is in the Aster/Daisy Family.

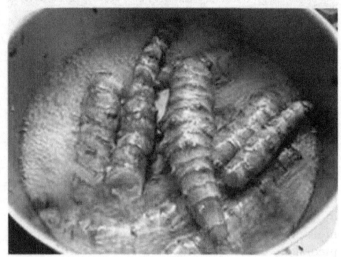

Jerusalem Artichoke, Paul Fenwick, CC SA 3.0

Identification: Jerusalem artichoke grows up to 10 feet (3 meters) tall. Rough, hairy leaves can be found opposing each other on the upper part of the stem, while lower leaves are alternate. The lower leaves are larger, up to a foot long. Higher leaves are smaller and narrow. Yellow flowers are a composite of 60 or more disc florets in the flower head, surrounded by 10 to 20 ray florets. Small sunflower seeds grow on the disc. The flower head grows up to 4 inches (10 cm) in diameter. The edible tubers are elongated, up to 4 inches (10 cm) long and 2 inches (5 cm) in diameter. Their appearance

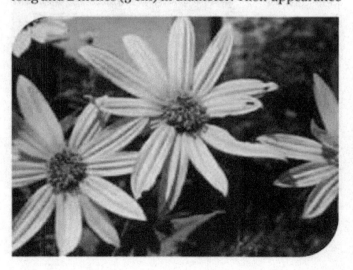

resembles ginger root. However, the color can vary from white to pale brown, or even red or purple.

Edible Use: The cooked root tuber is eaten as a vegetable and tastes similar to an artichoke, hence the name. I use the tubers as a substitute for potatoes; they have a sweeter, nuttier flavor.

They can be eaten raw, made into flour, pickled, or cooked. For some people, Jerusalem artichokes cause flatulence and gastric pain, so watch for gastric problems when Jerusalem artichokes are first introduced to the diet.

Medicinal Use: Jerusalem artichoke's medicinal action is due to its high concentration of inulin. It is one of the best sources of this valuable component available. To use Jerusalem artichoke for medicinal purposes, simply include it as a vegetable in the daily diet.

Diabetes: Fresh Jerusalem artichokes are approximately 76% inulin (not to be confused with insulin), which helps regulate blood sugar levels in diabetics. During storage, the inulin is converted to fructose, giving the tuber a sweet taste. Tubers grown in warm weather have higher insulin levels than those in colder regions, but all can be used to help control blood sugar in diabetes.

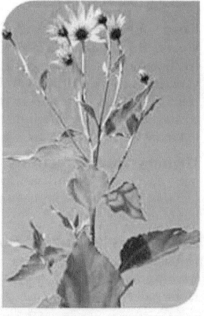

Jerusalem Artichoke Flowers, Paul Fenwick, CC by SA 3.0

Digestive Problems: Jerusalem artichokes are useful as a prebiotic fiber to help increase beneficial gut flora. They also stimulate stomach secretions that help control indigestion, dyspepsia, and slow digestion. However, Jerusalem artichokes do cause gas and intestinal pain in some people.

Enhances the Immune System: Jerusalem artichokes have immune-enhancing properties. They increase the body's defense mechanisms against viruses and bacteria, and they help increase the deployment of white blood cells to areas of infection.

Harvesting: Dig up the roots in autumn or leave them in the ground over the winter to harvest in the spring. Store them in high humidity to prevent them from wilting and softening. Tubers left in the ground will sprout in the spring. The tubers bruise easily and lose moisture quickly, so I usually prefer to leave them in the ground and harvest them when needed.

Warning: Jerusalem Artichokes can cause digestive distress and excessive gas in some people.

Lady's Thumb, *Polygonum persicaria* or *Persicaria maculosa*

Lady's thumb, also known as smartweed, heart's ease, spotted knotweed, or redshank, is a broadleaf weed that is often found growing in large clumps. It grows in disturbed wet soil across North America. It is in the Polygonaceae (Buckwheat/Knotweed) Family.

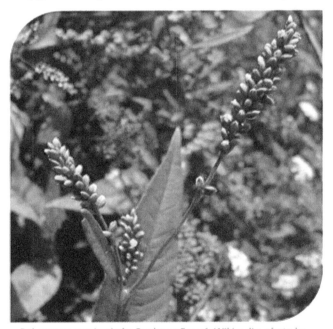
Polygonum persicaria by Bouba at French Wikipedia, photo by Bouba, CC-BY-SA-3.0-migrated

Identification: Lady's thumb grows from 1 to 3 feet tall (0.3 meters to 0.9 meters) and is an erect plant. The 2 to 6-inch-long (5 cm to 17.5 cm) leaves are alternate, narrow, and lance-shaped with wavy edges. They usually, but not always, have a dark green to purple spot in the middle. Leaves may be hairless or covered sparsely with small stiff hairs. Leaf nodes are surrounded by a thin papery membrane that wraps around the stem. The small, dark pink, (rarely white)

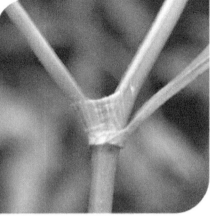
Stem of Lady's Thumb, Martin Olsson, CC by SA 3.0

flowers are densely packed in 1-inch (2.5 cm) spiked terminal clusters. They spike open, while those of the pale look-alike smartweed remain closed (pale smartweed also lacks the purple leaf smudge). Each bloom is approximately 1/8 inch (0.35 cm) across with five petals. Fruits are brown to black and glossy. They have three sides and are egg-shaped. Each fruit contains one tiny seed.

Edible Use: The leaves and young shoots can be eaten raw or cooked. Gather young leaves and sprouts in the spring to mid-summer. As they mature, they become more peppery and less palatable. The seeds are also edible, but they are rather small and require a lot of work to harvest enough to make a serving.

Medicinal Use: Use as a tea, decoction, or by applying the leaves directly to the skin.

Stomach Pains: For stomach pain and digestive upset, drink a leaf tea.

Skin Ailments: Lady's thumb is a rubefacient, and thus increases blood circulation at the skin's surface, supporting healing. It is also an astringent. Use for poison ivy, poison oak, skin rashes, and other skin ailments. Rub the crushed leaves on the skin or put a poultice on the surface of the skin.

Arthritis: For arthritic pain, soak in a tub of warm water containing a decoction of lady's thumb. The decoction can also be mixed with flour to form a wet poultice to help relieve painful joints.

Lamb's Quarter, Goosefoot, *Chenopodium album*

Lamb's Quarter is also called chualar, pigweed, and also goosefoot from the shape of its leaves. Lamb's quarter likes moist areas and grows near streams, rivers, in open meadows, and wet forest clearings. It is found throughout the world. It is a member of the Amaranthaceae (Amaranth) Family.

Identification: Lamb's quarter looks like a dusty weed from a distance. The alternate toothed leaves are light green on top and whitish on the bottom. They are somewhat diamond-shaped or shaped like a goosefoot.

The leaf surface is waxy and rain and dew rolls right off the leaves. Each leaf grows up to 4 inches (10 cm) long and the entire plant is usually 2 to 4 feet (0.6 to 1.3m) tall. Lamb's quarter produces tiny green flower clusters on top of spikes in summer. The flowers are densely packed together along the main stem and upper branches.

Each flower has five green sepals with no petals. Its seeds are small, round, and flattened. Branches are angular, somewhat ridged, and striped with pink, purple, or yellow. The stems are ribbed and are usually stained with purple or red.

Edible and Other Use: In the USA this plant is considered a weed; however, in some places, it is grown as a food crop. The young shoots, leaves, flowers, and seeds are all edible and can be used like spinach. Lamb's Quarter appears on my plate quite often. I find it a delicious and nutritious addition to my salads and even grow it in my garden.

It has a strong, slightly sweet flavor. The plant does contain oxalic acid so smaller quantities are recommended when eaten raw. The seeds of this herb should be cooked or soaked in water before use. The soaked seeds can also be ground into a powder to use as a flour. Lamb's quarter roots can be crushed to make a mild soap substitute as it contains saponins.

Medicinal Use: The plant is very nutritious and contains a rich source of vitamins A, B-2, C, and Niacin and minerals like calcium, iron, and phosphorus. It has been used as a vegetable to treat scurvy and other nutritional diseases.

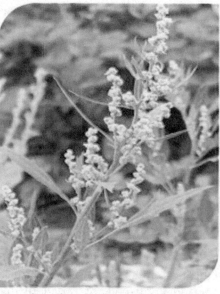
Goosefoot, Photo by Rasbak, CC by SA 3.0

Soothing Burns: Use a poultice made of the leaves to soothe burns. Bruise the leaves and place them on the burned area. Apply a clean cloth over them and leave in place for a few hours.

Skin Irritations, Eczema, Bites, Itching and Swelling: A poultice made from simmered, fresh lamb's quarter leaves can be applied to treat minor skin irritations, itching, rashes, and swelling. It soothes the skin, reduces inflammation (it is an anti-inflammatory), and helps the skin heal. If fresh herbs are not available, use a compress made with Lamb's Quarters Decoction. For internal inflammation, lightly steam the leaves and eat them as a vegetable.

Digestive Issues and as a Mild Laxative: Its leaves are loaded with fiber. This fiber makes it very effective in preventing and treating constipation. Cooked leaves loosen the stools and increase bowel movements.

Taken internally, lamb's quarter relieves stomachaches and digestive complaints, including colic. You can eat the cooked leaves and stems while eating beans to relieve the gas caused by them. Even easier, cook the leaves and stems in the pot with the beans.

Relieves Pain from Arthritis and Gout: Apply a poultice made from fresh, simmered lamb's quarter leaves directly on the skin above the inflammation and pain to treat arthritis and gout. When fresh leaves are not available, use Lamb's Quarters Decoction on the skin as a wash or in a compress.

Dental Health and Tooth Decay:
Use a Lamb's Quarter Decoction to treat tooth decay and bad breath. Apply a drop or two of the decoction directly onto the tooth or rinse the mouth with the liquid. It calms inflammation and pain. You can also chew on the raw leaves.

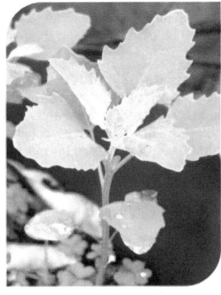

Young goosefoot, 6th Happiness, CC by SA 3.0

Colds, Flu and General Illness: Serve lamb's quarters as a vegetable when people have a cold or flu with respiratory problems. It functions as a mild analgesic to relieve body aches, induces perspiration to bring down fevers, and acts as an expectorant to help the body get rid of excess mucous. It also has anti-asthmatic properties and contains Vitamin C.

Harvesting: Break off or prune the top two inches (5 cm) of shoots. The tops are more tender and less bitter. Choose plants from secluded places, away from roadways, industrial areas, and waste sites where they may pick up high levels of nitrates and other toxins. Wash the leaves before use.

Warning: Lamb's quarter is an edible plant that has very little risk when used in moderate amounts. However, the plant does contain saponins in small quantities. Saponins are broken down by the cooking process. Like many green, leafy vegetables, it also contains oxalate crystals, which are not recommended in large amounts for people susceptible to kidney stones.

Recipes. Lamb's Quarter Decoction: Shred fresh lamb's quarter leaves into small pieces and pack into a cup to measure. Place the leaves in a pot and add an equal measure of water. Bring to a boil and simmer for 10 minutes. Once the herbs are wilted, add more water only if needed to cover the herbs. Cool the decoction and strain out the leaves. Keep in the refrigerator for up to 3 days. (The leaves can be eaten if desired).

Lavender, *Lavandula angustifolia*

Common lavender belongs to the Lamiaceae (Mint) Family. It is also known as garden lavender, common lavender, narrow-leaved lavender, true lavender, or English lavender.

Identification: Common lavender grows 1 to 3 feet (0.3m to 0.9meters) high in gardens. It has an irregular, erect, bluntly-quadrangular and multi-branched stem that is covered with a yellowish-grey bark, which comes off in flakes. It is covered with fine hairs.

The leaves of lavender are opposite, entire, and linear. When young, they are white with dense hairs on both surfaces. When full grown, leaves are 1 1/2 inch-long (3.75 cm) and green, with scattered hairs on the upper leaf surface. The flowers grow in terminating, blunt spikes from young shoots on long stems. The spikes are composed of whorls of flowers, each having 6 to 10 flowers, and the lower whorls are more distant from

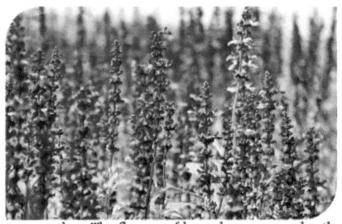

one another. The flowers of lavender are very shortly stalked. The calyx of lavender is tubular and ribbed, purple-grey in color, 5-toothed (one tooth is longer than the others) and hairy. The shining oil glands amongst the hairs are visible through a lens. Most of the oil yielded by the flowers is contained in the glands on the calyx. The two-lipped corolla is a beautiful bluish-violet color. It mostly lives and prefers dry grassy slopes amongst rocks, in exposed, usually parched, hot rocky situations often on calcareous soils. While not native to North America, it cultivates easily and spreads wild in many warm, dry areas.

Edible Use: Several parts of lavender are edible including the leaves, flowering tips, and petals. They can be used as a condiment in salads and make a nice tea. Fresh lavender flowers can be added to ice creams, jams, and vinegars as a flavoring. Oil from the flowers is also used as a food flavoring.

Medicinal Use: Medicinal uses are anti-anxiety, antiseptic, antispasmodic, bile-producing, diuretic, nervine, reduces gas, sedative, and stimulant.

Aromatherapy: Lavender is an important relaxing herb, having a soothing and relaxing effect upon the nervous system. In most cases, all that is required is to

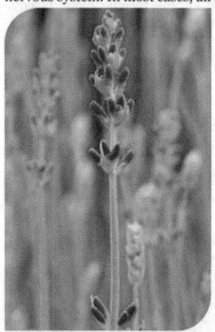

breathe in the aroma from the oil. This relaxes the body, relieves stress, calms the nervous system, and eases headaches. The same effects can be achieved by adding whole fresh or dried flowers to the bathwater or placing the flowers under the pillowcase at bedtime. I add it to my First Aid Salve so that the aroma is calming to anyone injured who is using the salve.

Aches and Pains: Its relaxing effects extend to the muscular system as well. A massage with lavender oil can calm throbbing muscles, relieve arthritis pain, ease and help heal sprains and strains, and relieve backaches and lumbago pain. The oil also contains analgesic compounds that help ease the pain from muscle related stress and injuries.

Kills Lice and Their Nits and Insect Repellent: The essential oil of lavender nourishes the hair, gives it a nice shine, and makes it smell wonderful. It also helps keep the hair free from lice.

Use the essential oil, diluted with a carrier oil such as coconut oil or olive oil, to coat the scalp and hair

completely. Give it an hour to soak in and do its magic. Then wash away the oil and use your nit comb. From this point forward, add a drop or two of lavender oil to your shampoo or rinse water to keep lice away. Lavender oil is also an excellent, good-smelling insect repellent.

Respiratory Problems: Lavender essential oil is an excellent treatment for respiratory problems of all kinds. This can include simple, everyday problems like colds, the flu, sore throats, coughs, and sinus congestion. It can also be used for more difficult and chronic respiratory issues like asthma, laryngitis, bronchitis, whooping cough, and tonsillitis.

Apply it topically to the skin on the chest, neck, and under the nose where it will be easily breathed; or add it to a vaporizer or a pot of steaming water. The nicely scented steam opens the air passages and loosens phlegm while it kills the germs that cause the infection.

Urinary Tract Infections, Cystitis and Retained Fluids: The diuretic effects of lavender help it to flush the body from excess fluids and toxins and relieve swellings that may be present. As the fluid is removed, the oil also exerts an antibiotic influence, which kills any underlying infection, and it removes toxins that may also be causing problems.

Lowering Blood Pressure: Removing excess fluids help lower the blood pressure and reduce swellings of all kinds, and the relaxing effects of the lavender help get rid of stresses that may be contributing to the problem.

Harvesting: I usually go out looking for Lavender when the weather is dry and there is no wind. The morning and evening are particularly favorable to gathering flowers because many of the oils are dissipated during the heat of the day. Cut lavender stems are cut at the base of the plant.

Recipes. Lavender Tea: To make lavender tea, start with one teasapoon of dried lavender flowers or one tablespoon of fresh lavender flowers. Place in a tea pot and cover with one cup of boiling water. Cover the tea pot to keep it warm and allow the tea steep for 10 to 15 minutes to absorb the medicinal qualities. Strain it, and drink warm several times daily.

Lavender Tincture: Ingredients: 1½ cups of chopped lavender flowers, stems, and leaves, 1-pint (500 ml)100 proof vodka or brandy. Place the lavender in a glass jar and cover with vodka. Seal the jar tightly and place it in a cool dark place to brew. Allow the tincture to steep for 4 to 6 weeks, shaking the jar daily. Strain the tincture through a coffee filter. Store it in a cool, dark place for up to 3 years.

Lavender Oil Distillation: Distillation equipment: a still OR small pressure cooker, glass tubing, tinned copper tubing, flexible hose, tub of cold water, collection vessel, thermometer. You'll need lavender flowers, stems, and leaves chopped fine or ground, water to cover the herbs. If you have a commercially available still, follow the instructions for steam distillation of essential oil. Otherwise, proceed with my directions to use a pressure cooker for steam distillation. Build a cooling coil out of tin-plated copper tubing. Wrap the tubing around a can or other cylinder to shape it for cooling the oil. Use a small piece of flexible hose to connect the copper tubing to the pressure cooker relief valve.

The steam will rise through the valve and flow into the copper tubing to cool. Bend the copper tubing as needed to place the coil into a pan or a tub of cold water. Cut a small hole in the bottom side of the tub for the copper tubing to exit the tub. Seal the exit hole with a stopper or silicone sealer. The tubing now runs down from the pressure cooker, into the cooling tub, out of the tub into your collection vessel. Place the chopped flowers, stems, and leaves into the pressure cooker. Add water as needed to cover the herbs and fill the pressure cooker to a level of 2 to 3 inches (5 cm to 7.5 cm). Heat the pressure cooker gently and watch for the oil to begin collecting in the collection vessel.

The oil will begin to distill near the boiling point of the water, but before the water boils. Watch for oil production. Monitor the still to make sure it does not boil dry. Collect the distillate until it becomes clear or until most of the water has distilled. The cloudy oil and water mixture indicate oil in the distillate. Once the distillate is clear, it contains only water, and the distillation is finished. Transfer the distilled oil to a dark glass bottle with a tight lid for storage. Lavender Essential Oil is much gentler than most other essential oils and can be safely applied directly to the skin as an antiseptic to help heal wounds and burns.

Leeks, *Allium porrum*

Leeks belong to the Alliaceae (Onion) Family. They are eaten as a vegetable and are quite tasty roasted or in soups. The flavor is mild compared to most members of the onion family.

Identification: Leeks grow from a compressed stem with leaves wrapped in overlapping layers and fanning out at the top. Commercial leeks are white at the base, caused by cultivation methods of piling soil at the base of the stem.

Wild leeks will not exhibit this blanching. Shallow, fibrous roots grow from the stem plate, and the plant grows upward reaching approximately 3 feet (0.9meters). If left in the ground, it produces a large umbel of flowers in the second year. The flowers produce small black, irregular seeds. The flower appears from July to August and has both male and female parts. It is tolerant to frost.

Edible Use: The leek is used extensively around the world as a vegetable and as a flavoring. It contains vitamins, antioxidants, and minerals and is low in calories and high in fiber.

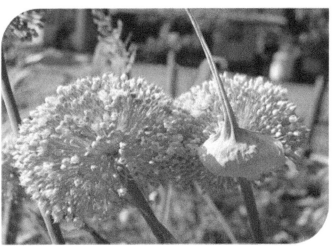

Leek Flower Heads, Photo by Derek Ramsey (Ram-Man) - Own work, CC by SA 2.5

Medicinal Use. Heart Disease, High Blood Pressure, Lowering Cholesterol: Leeks are beneficial to the heart and circulatory system in a number of ways. They contain enzymes that help reduce the harmful cholesterols in the body while increasing the beneficial HDL cholesterols.

They also relax the blood vessels, arteries, and veins, reducing the blood pressure and they reduce the formation of clots and help break down existing clots. In

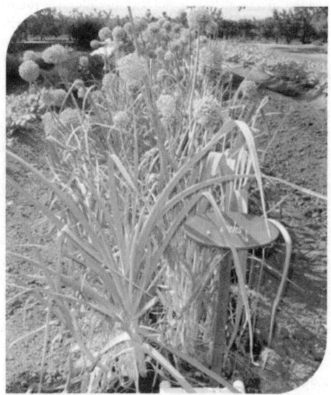

these ways, they reduce the chances of developing coronary heart disease, peripheral vascular diseases, and strokes.

Consuming leeks on a regular basis conveys these beneficial properties.

Stabilize Blood Sugar Levels: Leeks help the body maintain a steady blood sugar level by helping the body metabolize sugars. Leeks also contain nutrients that benefit blood sugar levels. Diabetics and pre-diabetics should eat leeks regularly as part of their healthy diet.

Anti-Bacterial, Anti-Viral, and Anti-Fungal Properties: Eating leeks regularly and often during infections helps your body fight these infections and eliminate them from the body.

Leeks have anti-microbial properties similar to those of garlic and onions that help the body fight internal and external infections.

Eat an extra portion of leeks with meals when fighting infections. For external infections, chop the leeks finely and use them as a poultice on infected tissue.

Prevents Cancer: Plants in the Alliaceae family have multiple cancer-fighting properties, and leeks are included. Eating leeks on a regular basis reduces the chances of prostate and colon cancers. People who eat a lot of leeks also have fewer ovarian cancers.

Eat Leeks During Pregnancy: Leeks contain high levels of folate, which is beneficial for the developing fetus and prevents several different birth defects of the brain and spinal cord.

Anemia: Leeks are also high in iron and therefore beneficial for treating iron deficiency anemia. They also contain significant levels of vitamin C, which helps iron absorption in the body.

Gout, Arthritis, and Urinary Tract Inflammation: Arthritis, gout, and urinary tract problems benefit from the anti-inflammatory and antiseptic properties of leeks to treat these diseases.

High doses of leeks are best, so I recommend eating several servings daily or drinking the juice of the vegetable.

Regular Bowel Movements: The high concentrations of both soluble and insoluble dietary fiber in leeks help the function of the intestinal tract. They facilitate digestion and reduce bloating and associated pain.

Whole Body Cleanse: Drinking leek juice regularly helps cleanse the body of toxins and waste products.

Harvesting: Harvest when the stalks are about an inch (2.5 cm) wide, usually in late summer. In some areas they over-winter and can be harvested in early spring or even year-round.

Warning: Leeks contain oxalates, which may crystalize in the body to cause kidney stones and gravel in the gallbladder.

Lemon Balm, *Melissa officinalis*

Lemon Balm is a perennial member of the Lamiaceae (Mint) Family with valuable healing properties. Sometimes called common balm or balm mint, it is naturalized in North America. I love the lemony scent that is released when I walk through a patch of lemon balm.

Identification: Lemon balm is a mint with shiny bright green leaves and a lemony scent. It may grow to 3 feet (0.9m) in height and is easy to cultivate in the garden. Its appearance is similar to mint or catnip, but the lemon scent is intense when leaves are disturbed or crushed. The leaves are small heart shapes with scalloped edges and a slightly crinkled surface. Small flowers are usually white to yellow but can be pink or purple.

Edible Use: The leaves are edible and often used to make tea and as a flavoring ingredient. It makes a delicious tea for medicinal or culinary use and is enhanced by the use of raw honey to sweeten it.

Medicinal Use: Lemon balm leaves are often used as a tea, extract, tincture, oil, or ointment.

Relieves Anxiety and Insomnia: Lemon balm

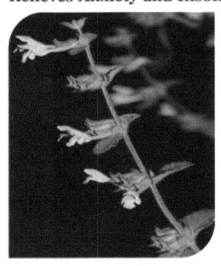

acts to reduce anxiety and helps people get better sleep. It calms the body and improves mood and intellectual performance in children and adults without negative effects. For reducing the effects of sleep disorders, especially during menopause, try a combination of lemon balm and valerian.

Lemon Balm Flowers, Gideon Pisanty, CC BY 3.0

Lemon balm helps stop the constant flow of anxious thoughts. It also helps with ADHD and mild depression.

Mind Calming and Clear Thinking: Lemon balm seems to calm the mind and allows people to

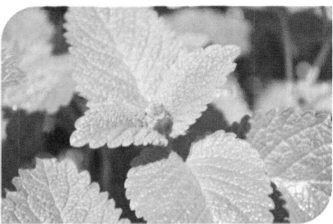

think more clearly. It increases mental alertness and promotes a positive attitude.

Anti-Viral Effects: Herpes, Cold Sores, and Shingles: Lemon balm is known as an anti-viral and is effective against herpes and cold sores when applied directly to the skin. It acts against the herpes simplex virus and when used regularly, people report fewer outbreaks and fast healing of existing lesions. It also gives relief of symptoms like itching and burning. Try lemon balm essential oil or lemon balm ointment on herpes and cold sores. Apply several times daily or as needed. For shingles take a tincture internally as well as apply topically to the affected area.

PMS Symptoms: Lemon balm reduces symptoms of PMS, including cramping, anxiety, and headaches. It works well for PMS in teenage and adult women. It is an anti-spasmodic.

Protects the Heart: Lemon balm, used regularly, lowers triglycerides and improves cholesterol synthesis. It controls heart palpitations and lowers blood pressure while protecting the heart. It controls the electrical pulses that drive heart palpitations, tachycardia, and arrhythmias.

Protects the Liver: Lemon balm protects the liver from some of the negative effects of the American diet. It supports the liver's production of antioxidants and helps detox the liver.

Antibacterial and Antifungal: Lemon Balm oil has a high level of antibacterial and antifungal activity. It is particularly active against *Candida* yeast infections. Use lemon balm oil, tincture or extract twice a day.

Diabetes: Lemon balm oil, tincture and extract are effective in preventing and treating diabetes. It helps control blood sugar levels and protects the body against the oxidative stress caused by diabetes.

Anti-Inflammatory and Antioxidant: Lemon balm oil acts as an anti-inflammatory and antioxidant. It reduces inflammation in the body, protecting against disease and reducing pain.

Fights Cancer: Lemon balm has been shown to kill some cancer cell lines, including breast cancer, colorectal cancer, and aggressive brain cancers. Lemon balm supports the body in fighting the cancer cells.

Regulates the Thyroid: Hyperthyroidism, or an over-active thyroid benefits from the regular consumption of lemon balm. People with Grave's disease or other over-active thyroid problems find that the oil, tincture or extract helps regulate thyroid-binding problems.

Aids in Digestion: Lemon balm extract has a protective effect on the gastrointestinal system and prevents gastric ulcers. It aids digestion and is useful in treating constipation as well as colic.

Alzheimer's Disease and Dementia: Lemon balm extract is believed to reduce damage from plaque forming proteins in Alzheimer's disease. Regular administration of lemon balm extract increases cognitive function over time and reduces agitation in Alzheimer's patients.

The therapy is not a cure, but is observed to slow progression and help promote mild improvements. As an anti-oxidant it may help protect the brain from neuro-degeneration and oxidative damage.

Lemon Balm also improves memory and problem solving in people of all ages and health levels including Alzheimer's patients.

Heals Skin and Reduces Signs of Aging: People who use lemon balm on their skin report that it reduces wrinkles and fine lines giving the skin a more youthful appearance. It is particularly beneficial in supporting the skin against minor blemishes and infections.

Harvesting: Left alone, lemon balm may take over the garden. Several bouts of pruning keep the plant in check. Clip off stems or remove individual leaves for

drying on screens, in a dehydrator, or hand them in bunches to dry. I like to harvest just before the plant flowers (early to late summer).

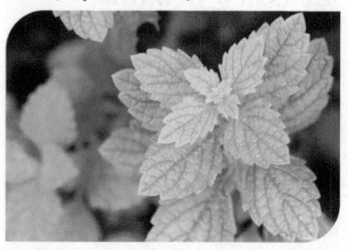

Warning: Lemon balm is considered safe for most people, but should not be used by people on thyroid medication or with underactive thyroids (Hypothyroidism).

Consult a medical profession before using lemon balm regularly if you are pregnant or nursing. Possible side effects include headache, nausea, bloating, gas, indigestion, dizziness, and allergic reactions. Consult a doctor if you are taking other medications or planning surgical treatments.

Recipes. Lemon Balm Tea: You will need: 1 tablespoon fresh lemon balm leaves or 1t dried and 1 cup boiling water. Tear the leaves into small pieces and put into a tea ball, or filter the leaves after brewing.

Pour boiling water over the tea leaves or ball and allow to infuse for 5 minutes. Keep the pot or cup covered while brewing and drinking to retain the beneficial aromatics.

Lemon Balm Extract/Tincture: Ingredients: 1-pint (500ml) jar with a tight-fitting lid, 80 proof or higher vodka or another alcoholic beverage. Wash and dry the leaves and crush them lightly.

Fill the jar 3/4 full with leaves and pour the vodka, filling the jar completely. Cap and store in a cool, dark place, shaking periodically. After 4 to 6 weeks, strain and label.

Lemon Thyme, *Thymus citriodorus*

Lemon thyme is also called citrus thyme. It is easy to recognize lemon thyme by its aroma and flavor, which are both very much like lemon. Even better than the smell are the relaxing benefits and medicinal value of the herb. It is in the Lamiaceae (Mint) Family.

Identification: Lemon thyme is an evergreen perennial that grows as a mat on the ground. It grows to a height of 4 inches (10 cm) and spreads to over a foot away. Its appearance and growth habit is close to that of English thyme.

The leaves are shiny-green with a pale-yellow border around the margins. Some plants have more lemon-yellow leaves or green leaves with pale yellow splotches. The plant produces flowers in mid to late

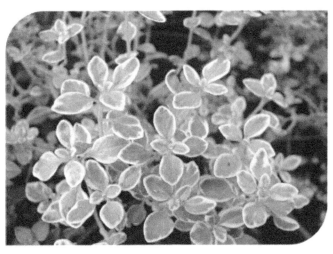

Lemon Thyme, Forest & Kim Starr, CC by SA 3.0

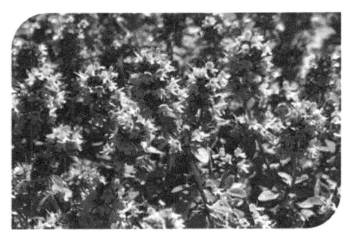

Lemon Thyme flowers, Kor!An (Андрей Корзун), CC by SA 3.0

summer. Flowers may vary from pink to lavender and attract butterflies and bees.

Edible Use: Lemon thyme is used widely in cooking to flavor chicken, fish, and vegetable dishes and to make a relaxing tea.

Medicinal Use: Immune Function: Lemon Thyme Tea is a relaxing drink that is effective in the treatment of infections and boosting the immune system. It makes a good tonic for regular use.

Viral, Bacterial, and Fungal Infections: The anti-microbial properties of lemon thyme make it effective in the fight against most bacterial, fungal, and viral diseases.

Respiratory Problems, Asthma, and Releasing Congestion: Lemon thyme contains many different beneficial compounds for general health and for respiratory health. It is an anti-microbial and a decongestant.

It opens the airways to help asthmatics breathe better and to allow phlegm and other mucous to be released from the body.

Aromatherapy for Asthma: Asthmatics find relief by placing a small pillow filled with dried lemon thyme under their regular pillow. Sleeping on this pillow releases the oils that open the airways and induce better sleep.

Warning: Lemon thyme causes allergic reactions in highly allergic people. Do not give lemon thyme tea during pregnancy or while nursing.

Lemon Thyme Tea: You'll need 1/2 teaspoon of dried lemon thyme or 1 teaspoon of fresh lemon thyme leaves, 1 cup boiling water and honey, optional. Pour the boiling water over the lemon thyme leaves and allow the tea to steep for 5 to 10 minutes.

Strain the tea and drink warm. Add honey as desired for sweetening. Drink two to three cups daily.

Lemon Verbena, *Aloysia triphylla*

Oh, how I love lemon verbena. I love to crush a stalk in my hand and breathe in the fragrance and flavor. It immediately lifts my mood and soothes away the stresses of the day. The herb is highly aromatic with an herbaceous lemony scent. It is in the Verbenaceae (Verbena) Family. It is not native but is easily cultivated in the garden.

Identification: Lemon verbena is readily identified by its scent and the plant growth. It grows to a height of 6 to 15 feet (1.8m to 4.5m) in good soil. It has thin, pointed leaves that are about 3 to 4 inches (7.5 cm to 10 cm) in length. The leaves are shiny and coarse to the touch. The flowers are light purple and grouped on the stems. They appear throughout the summer.

Edible Use: Lemon verbena leaves are useful as a flavoring or as an addition to salads. It has a mild lemon flavor.

Medicinal Use: Use lemon verbena leaves and flowers internally in the form of an herbal tea and externally as a poultice, oil, or wash.

Bronchial Congestion: Use a tea made from lemon verbena to treat bronchial and nasal congestion. It loosens phlegm, acts as an expectorant, and calms the system. Do not use lemon verbena tea before driving or operating heavy machinery as it has a mild sedative effect.

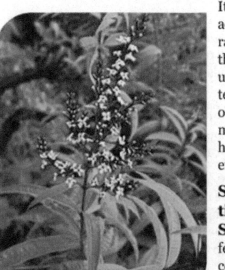

Lemon Verbena, H. Zell, CC by SA 3.0

Staph Infections of the Skin: Staph infections can become serious quickly if left untreated. It prevents the infection from spreading and kills the existing

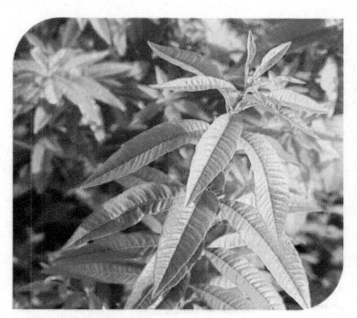

bacteria. For this purpose, use Lemon Verbena Leaf Tincture made with 80 proof alcohol, applied to the skin. When the extraction is not available, a poultice of freshly crushed lemon verbena is applied (note that Usnea also works well on *Staphylococcus*).

Arthritis, Bursitis, and Joint Pain: Peoples with joint pain find significant relief from taking lemon verbena tea. It takes time for the effects to build, but over a period of two to three months of taking the tea twice daily, people report that joint pain is gradually reduced and significant improvement is gained.

Digestive Issues: Try Lemon Verbena Tea for digestive problems as it has a soothing effect on the digestive system. It relieves indigestion and calms the stomach and intestinal spasms to relieve cramping and bloating. Try drinking a cup of tea after meals.

Calms Anxiety: For severe anxiety, try Lemon Verbena Tea. It soothes the nervous system, relieves stress, and lifts the mood.

Harvesting: Lemon verbena likes rich soil and plenty of sunlight. I collect the leaves throughout the year, but I prefer to pick as many as possible before the herb blooms. Extra leaves are dried for future use and are equally beneficial in dried form.

Recipes. Lemon Verbena Tea: 1/4 cup lemon verbena leaves, fresh and crushed, 2 cups boiling water. Pour the boiling water over the herb and allow it to steep for 5 to 8 minutes. Strain and Drink 1 cup.

Lemon Verbena Tincture: Take fresh Lemon Verbena leaves and flowers, chopped, 80 proof vodka or other drinking alcohol and a jar with a tight-fitting lid. Add the lemon verbena to the jar, packing it about three quarters full.

Pour the vodka over the leaves and fill the jar, making sure all the leaves are covered. Cap the jar tightly and place it in a cool, dark place, such as a cupboard. Let the tincture steep for 6 to 8 weeks, shaking the jar daily. Pour the alcohol through a fine mesh sieve or a coffee filter to remove all the herb. Store the tincture in a cool, dark cupboard for up to 7 years.

Licorice Root, *Glycyrrhiza glabra*

Licorice root is an adaptogenic herb that thrives in USDA growing zones 6 through 11. It is well known for its strong candy flavor but is a valuable medicinal herb for treating many illnesses.

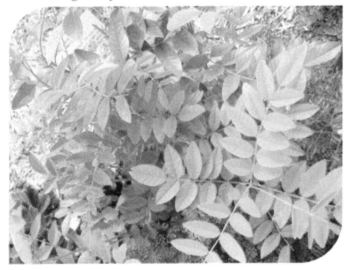

Photo By Gardenology.org, CC by SA 3.0

Glycyrrhiza glabra and Glycyrrhiza uralensis are medicinally similar, but here we are referring to Glycyrrhiza glabra. It is a member of the legume/pea family (Fabaceae).

Identification: Glycyrrhiza glabra grows to approximately 3 feet tall (0.9m). Its pinnate leaves are 3 to 6 inches long (7.5 – 15cm) with 9 to 17 leaflets each. The purple to pale blue flowers are about 1/2 inch long (1.25cm), growing in a loose inflorescence. In the fall the plant produces fruit in the form of an oblong pod, each of which contains several seeds. The root produces runners growing close to the surface.

Medicinal Use: The roots and leaves contain many types of compounds that are medically active: coumarins, triterpenoids, glabrene, and polyphenols. These compounds are antibacterial, antiviral, anti-inflammatory, and include natural steroid compounds.

Glycyrrhizin, one of the components of licorice root, can cause side-effects if overused or taken in large doses. Be aware of all side-effects and interactions before using licorice root.

You can also get deglycyrrhizinated licorice (DGL), which has the glycyrrhizin removed, thus preventing its side effects.

Leaky Gut Syndrome and Inflammation: Leaky gut, or intestinal permeability, is an inflammatory disease of the intestinal tract. Licorice root soothes the intestines and reduces inflammation in the gut and throughout the body.

Peptic Ulcers: Licorice root is effective against the Helicobacter pylori bacteria that cause peptic ulcers. The root kills the bacteria and helps heal the ulcers in most people.

Heartburn, Stomach Problems, and Acid Reflux: Licorice root has shown to be effective against indigestion heartburn, acid reflux, indigestion, stomach pain, and nausea.

Fertility Problems, PMS, and Menopause Symptoms: Licorice root has an estrogen-like effect in women, due to the compound glabrene, which is a phytoestrogen. It has been shown to help menstrual and fertility problems. When used as a hormone replacement therapy, it reduces hot flashes and other symptoms of menopause due to the compounds liquiritigenin and glabrene.

Cancer: Licorice root may aid in the treatment of prostate and breast cancers. Research is still in progress on the use of licorice in cancer treatment, but the early results are promising.

Hepatitis C: Glycyrrhizin is an anti-viral and anti-inflammatory. It may act against the virus causing hepatitis C and helps reduce long-term liver damage from the disease. Herbalists use glycyrrhizin to treat chronic hepatitis C that does not respond to traditional treatments.

Immune System, Antiviral, Antioxidant: Licorice has proven antiviral, antibacterial, and antioxidant effects, boosting the work of the immune system. As an antiviral, it helps prevent diseases such as hepatitis C, HIV, and Influenza.

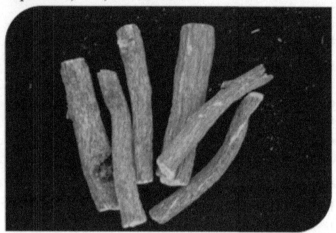

The Common Cold, Cough, and Sore Throats: In addition to its antiviral and anti-bacterial benefits, licorice root also acts as an expectorant, loosening and expelling mucus from the throat and lungs.

It is soothing and anti-inflammatory, which helps relieve the symptoms of sore throats. Use licorice root or leaves in tea, syrups, or to make cough drops for use against sore throats. It can also be used as a gargle.

Respiratory Issues: Licorice is useful in treating respiratory problems. It helps the body produce and expel mucus, which keeps the respiratory system clean and functioning properly. Used for COPD as well.

Treats Eczema, Skin Rashes: Licorice acts as a hydrocortisone to alleviate eczema, cellulitis, and folliculitis. Its anti-inflammatory benefits also help reduce swelling and irritation in skin conditions. Use licorice topically in a cleansing tea or in lotions or gels to relieve itching, redness, scaling, and inflammation caused by eczema or other skin problems.

Harvesting: Licorice is a perennial deciduous plant that requires three to four years to grow roots mature enough for harvest. Harvest the leaves throughout the spring through fall. Wait until the licorice roots are 3 to 4 years old before harvest. Young roots are too small to be of use.

Recipes. Liquid Extract: Licorice extract is a common form of licorice, it is used as a sweetener in candies and some beverages.

Limit your use of licorice extract to 30 mg/ml of glycyrrhizic acid. Higher doses can cause side-effects.

Licorice Root Powder: Licorice root powder is useful as is for treating skin problems or for use in capsules as an oral supplement. Combine it with a gel or lotion base to make a topical ointment or lotion for treating skin problems.

Licorice Leaf Tea: Use dried and crushed licorice leaves as a tea to promote health of the digestive and respiratory tract. Use 1 teaspoon of crushed leaves per 1 cup of boiling water.

DGL Licorice: DGL licorice is a commercial form of licorice with the glycyrrhizin removed. It is considered a safer form of licorice root and is particularly recommended for long term use. DGL is available commercially.

Warning: Long-term use of licorice root or high doses can have serious side effects. Most of the side effects are due to the presence of glycyrrhizin, so using DGL licorice reduces the risks.

Watch for these symptoms: low levels of potassium in the body, hypokalemia, muscle weakness, fluid retention and swelling, metabolism abnormalities, high blood pressure, heart rhythm irregularities, erectile dysfunction, potential drug interactions.

Pregnant or breastfeeding women should avoid licorice in all forms. Patients who are prone to hypertension should also avoid licorice root.

Also avoid use of licorice root if you have heart, liver, or kidney problems. Stop taking licorice root at least two weeks before surgery.

Lovage, *Levisticum officinale*

Lovage is native to Southern Europe, is easy to cultivate in the garden, and has naturalized in Eastern North America. It has a celery-like taste and is in the Apiaceae/ Umbelliferae (Celery/ Parsley /Carrot) Family.

Identification: Lovage grows to a height of 6 feet (1.8m). The plant is erect and its stems and leaves are hairless with a celery scent. Stems are thick and celery-like with additional flat lobed pinnate leaves. Yellow to greenish-yellow flowers, approximately 1 inch (2.5 cm) in diameter, bloom in late spring. Flowers grow in umbels 4 to 6 inches (10 cm to 15 cm) in diameter. Fruit matures in autumn, forming a 2-part seed.

Edible Use: Lovage is edible and a good addition wherever you would normally use celery. The taste is stronger than celery. The leaves can be used as a salad green or brewed into a tea. The seeds are used as a flavoring spice. Lovage is nutritionally healthy, adding B-complex vitamins and vitamin C to the diet.

Medicinal Use: Lovage root and leaves are effectively used in teas, decoctions, infusions, and tinctures. Leaves and roots can be added to bath water and foot soaks. All parts of the plant are medicinally active.

Soothes the Digestive Tract: Lovage seeds are effective in treating digestive problems and relieving intestinal gas. Simply chew the seeds for a quick remedy for digestive upsets, bloating, and gas.

Skin Conditions and Inflammations, Dermatitis, Acne, Psoriasis, Rashes: I prefer lovage root preparations for skin inflammations. The root pieces can be added to bathwater for a long soak or simmered in water to make a decoction for application to the affected areas. Lovage Leaf Oil Extract is also effective for applications to infections, wounds, and treating inflamed skin.

Reduces Inflammation and Irritation in the Body: Lovage is soothing throughout the body. It reduces irritation and inflammation that causes problems such as colitis, inflammatory bowel disease, and other diseases caused by inflammation.

Painful Joints: Painful joints from any cause, especially gout and arthritis, respond to treatment with lovage root both internally and externally. It reduces inflammation and lets the joints heal.

Respiratory Problems: Lovage roots and leaves help increase airflow and oxygen to the body. It loosens phlegm in the lungs and calms irritation.

Anti-Histamine: Lovage is a natural antihistamine that helps fight allergy symptoms. Quercetin, found in lovage, stops the release of histamines and soothes the irritations caused by the allergy. Use Lovage Tea internally and apply a decoction or oil for external relief of skin rashes or irritations.

Prevents Kidney Stones and Helps UTIs: For patients who have a history of kidney stones or urinary tract infections, try Lovage Root Tea or Tincture. It acts as a diuretic and increases the flow of urine without electrolyte loss. This flushing action helps prevent kidney stones from building in the kidneys.

Supports a Healthy Menstrual Cycle: Women can take Lovage Tea a day or two before their menstrual flow begins. It relieves cramping and bloating due to menstruation.

Harvesting: Harvest leaves before the plant flowers and use fresh or dry them for future use. Roots are harvested from plants that are 3 years old or older. Dig up the roots in autumn or early spring.

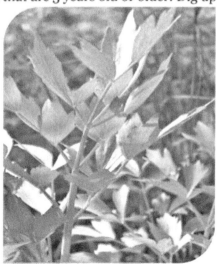

Recipes. Lovage Tea: You'll need one teaspoon of dried lovage or 1 tablespoon of fresh lovage leaves and 1 cup of boiling water. Pour the boiling water over the lovage and cover it to keep it warm. Let the tea steep for 10 to 15 minutes to absorb the medicinal qualities. Strain it, and drink warm several times daily.

Lovage Tincture: 1½ cups of chopped lovage root and leaves, 1 pint (500 ml) 80 proof vodka or brandy.

Place fresh or dried lovage in a glass jar and cover with vodka. Seal the jar tightly and place it in a cool dark place to brew. Allow the tincture to steep for 4 to 6 weeks, shaking the jar daily. Strain. Label and store it in a cool, dark place for up to 5 years.

Lungwort (Common) Plant, *Pulmonaria officinalis*

Common Lungwort is a beautiful little plant that grows as a groundcover in partial shade on the forest floor, reaching about a foot in height. It has several different names, including Bethlehem Sage, Jerusalem Cowslip, and Pulmonaire. Native to Europe it is easy to cultivate in the garden. It is in the Borage Family. It is different than Lungwort Lichen, also in this book. The leaves look slightly like a diseased lung, giving it the name lungwort and indicating its use in treating lung diseases.

Identification: The bright green leaves come to a point at one end. The leaf top is hairy and rough and leaves are covered with whitish or gray spots. Small bunches of flowers appear in spring. Each flower has 5 pinkish-blue or purple petals. Seeds ripen in late May or June.

Edible Use: The leaves of lungwort are edible both raw and cooked. They have a mucilaginous and hairy texture that makes them less appealing when uncooked.

Medicinal Use: Bronchitis, Asthma, Whooping Cough: Lungwort is effective in treating breathing problems such as chronic bronchitis, asthma, and whopping cough. The leaves are soothing and expectorant. Their mucilaginous properties make them useful in treating sore throats. Lungwort relieves bronchial inflammations of the airways and helps the body expel mucus. I like tea made from the leaves and flowers for this purpose. A recipe for Lungwort Tea is below. Alternatively, grind the dried flowers and leaves into a powder to use in capsule form or use a Lungwort Tincture.

Diarrhea and Digestive Complaints: The mucilaginous properties make the leaves effective in treating diarrhea and other digestive problems such as stomach pain, bloating, and indigestion.

Diuretic and Detoxify: Lungwort is a mild diuretic, and thus helps bloating and relieving the body of excess fluids. This is also beneficial for helping remove toxins from the body.

General Tonic for Health and Anti-Aging: Lungwort is rich in antioxidants and other compounds that are beneficial for health, slow down the aging pro-

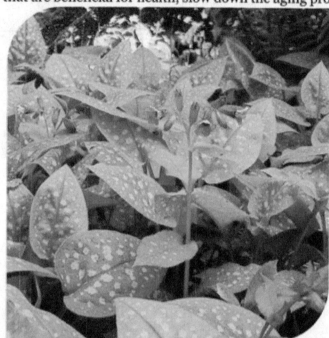

Lungwort with flowers, TeunSpaans, CC by SA 3.0

cess, and protect the body from free radical damage. It is also an excellent astringent.

Wounds, Cuts, Hemorrhoids, and Skin Diseases: Lungwort helps the skin heal from cuts and wounds and contributes to skin health. Apply it directly to the skin as a wash, compress, or poultice as needed for various skin conditions including burns, eczema, rashes, boils and ulcers, and to reduce and heal hemorrhoids. It is anti-inflammatory, anti-bacterial, and astringent.

Urinary Tract Infections, Cystitis, Kidney Problems: Because of its diuretic properties and antibacterial properties, Lungwort is beneficial in helping the body rid itself of excess fluids and aids the kidneys and urinary tract in the process. It treats urinary tract infections like cystitis (bladder infection), and helps expel toxins from the body.

Stops Bleeding: Taken internally as a powder or tea, lungwort is useful in reducing internal bleeding and excess menstrual bleeding. It can be applied directly to external wounds as a powder or whole leaf to bind a wound and stimulate clotting.

Ringworm: A Lungwort Decoction applied several times a day directly onto the skin will help with ringworm.

Harvesting: Harvest the flowers and leaves in the spring when the flowers first appear. Cut off the entire stem with leaves and flowers attached and tie them in bunches for hanging and drying.

Warning: Be cautious taking Lungwort if you are pregnant or breastfeeding. The plant has no known side effects, but caution is always warranted. Lungwort

can cause a skin rash in some people. Do not use Lungwort if you experience a rash or any adverse reaction.

Recipes. Lungwort Tea: 1 Tablespoon lungwort leaves and flowers, 1 cup boiling water, Raw honey, as desired for sweetness. Pour the boiling water over the leaves and flowers and allow it to steep for 15 minutes. Strain the tea and drink up to three cups daily. Raw honey helps alleviate the bitter flavor for some people.

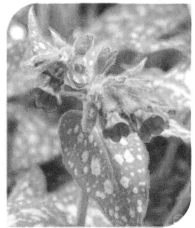

Lungwort Decoction for Wounds: 2 Tablespoons chopped, dried lungwort leaves and 1 cup boiling water. Make a strong tea, infusing the leaves in the boiling water for 20 minutes or until cool. Strain the decoction and use it to wash the skin and affected areas or apply it to a cloth and use as a compress.

Mallow,
Malva sylvestris

Mallow, also called high mallow, wood mallow, tree mallow, or cheeseweed, is a spreading herb that can be biennial. It is native to Europe and Asia but is naturalized throughout most of North America. This is a different plant than Marshmallow, also in this book. It is in the Malvaceae (Mallow) Family and looks similar to Hibiscus.

Identification: This plant grows from 3 to 10 feet (3m) high. Its branches are bare or covered with fine soft hairs. They have palmately lobed leaves that are dark green in color with long petioles. Leaves are 1 ½ to 2 inches (3.5 cm to 5 cm) across and are creased with 3 to 9 shallow lobes. Leaves on the stem are alternate. The leaves have a course feel but release mucilage when crushed. Purple-pink flowers bloom between May and August. Flowers grow in axillary clusters of 2 to 4 and form

along the main stem. They are about 2 inches (5 cm) in diameter with 5 dark, veined, notched petals. Flowers at the base of the stem open first. The fruit looks like

compressed disks or a cheese wheel, leading to the nickname "cheese flower." Ripe seeds are about ¼ inch (0.625 cm) in diameter and are brownish-green to brown in color.

Edible Use: All parts are edible raw or cooked and are mucilagenous. Leaves cook up much like okra. Cooked mallow roots can be beaten and used like egg whites in a meringue.

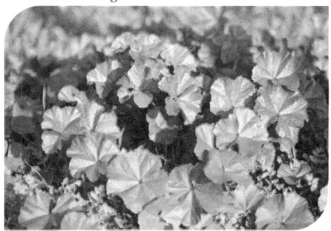

Medicinal Use: Mallow roots, leaves, seeds, and flowers are all used medicinally. The mucilage is very soothing and it is a good anti-inflammatory.

Soothes Irritated Mucous Membranes: Mallow Tea is helpful for cases of irritated mucous membranes. It soothes the lining of the respiratory tract and other mucus membranes for symptom relief of colds, coughs, bronchitis, emphysema, and asthma. It is also anti-inflammatory.

Burns, Bruising, Swelling and Other Topical Use: Mallow soothes inflamed tissue and works well for burns, dermatitis, and any type of swelling. It can be added to a bath or used on the skin.

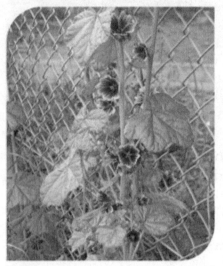

High Mallow, KENPEI, CC by SA 3.0

Anti-bacterial and Urinary Tract Infections: Leaf and flower tincture is antibacterial against *Staphylococcus*, *Streptococcus*, and *Enterococcus*. Best used in conjunction with stronger antibacterial herbs for UTIs and other infections. Mallow relieves the swelling and irritation of the urinary tract and helps promote healing.

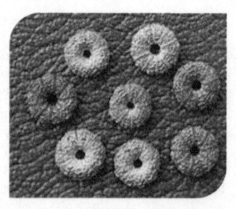

Nutlets or seeds, Qniemiec, CC by SA 3.0

Teething: Mallow Root Tea is safe for use with children and is a good antidote for teething pain and inflammation. Rub the tea onto the gums as often as needed.

Nausea, Stomach and Digestive Upsets: Mallow Leaf or Root Tea relieves nausea. It works well for stomach flu, ulcers, and other stomach upsets, soothing inflammation and promoting normal bowel function.

Recipes: Mallow Root Tea. 1 tablespoon of shredded or powdered mallow root, 1-pint (500 ml) of water. Bring the root and water to a boil and simmer for 5 to 10 minutes. Allow it to cool to drinking temperature and strain out the root. Drink 1 cup, warm or cold.

Marshmallow, *Althaea officinalis*

The common marshmallow plant is grown commercially for medicinal use, but it can be found in many places in the US growing wild. The roots were used to make the original marshmallow candy, unlike today's supermarket version, which are pure sugar. The plant grows in cool, moist places such as the grassy banks of lakes and streams and on the edges of marshes. I have seen it growing wild in many eastern and mid-western states. I grow it in my garden. It is in the Malvaceae (Mallow) Family.

Identification: Marshmallow is a green perennial with large white flowers that bloom from July to September. The plants grow to be from 4 to 6 feet (1.2m to 1.8m) tall and form clumps about 2 1/2 feet (0.8m) in diameter. The leaves vary in shape. Some are spearhead-shaped while others have three or five lobes or may be toothed. They are covered in a fine, velvety fuzz on both sides. The plant has many branchless stems covered in soft white hairs. The stems have sawtoothed projections. The flowers are somewhat trumpet-shaped, about 2 to 3 inches (5 cm to 7.5 cm) across and roughly 3 inches (7.5 cm) deep. The flowers produce seedpods that ripen in August to October, popping open to release small, flat black seeds.

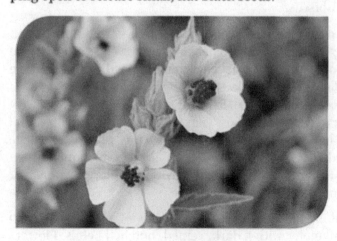

Edible Use: The leaves, flowers, root, and seeds are all edible. The roots contain a mucilage, which is sweet in flavor. Slice and boil the roots for 20 minutes, then remove from the liquid. Boil the remaining liquid again with sugar to taste and whip to make old-fashioned marshmallow candies.

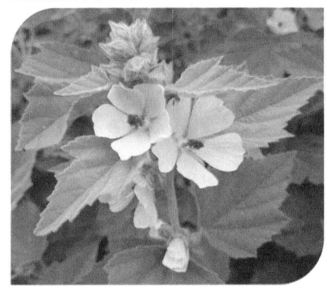

Medicinal Use: The roots, leaves, and flowers are used for medicinal treatments. They are especially valuable for treating problems with the mucous membranes.

Acid Indigestion, Peptic Ulcers, Leaky Gut, and Digestive Issues: I use the root of the marshmallow plant to treat stomach problems caused by excess stomach acid and for Leaky Gut. It is effective in neutralizing the acid and relieving symptoms. The root has a moderate laxative effect, which makes it useful in treating intestinal problems such as colitis, ileitis, irritable bowel syndrome, and diverticulitis. I also use it as an ingredient in my Leaky Gut Blend as it forms a protective layer around perforations in the gut.

Dry Coughs, Bronchitis, Bronchial Asthma, Congestion, and Pleurisy: Because marshmallow is so good at treating the membranes, it makes a good antidote for respiratory problems. It relieves the swelling and irritation of the mucous membrane and calms the respiratory system. It is not an expectorant.

Teething Pain: Young children can be given a piece of peeled fresh roots to chew on. The chewing stick relieves teething pain and has a mildly sweet taste. Watch closely and replace it before it gets so chewed that it could become a choking hazard.

Skin Irritations, Inflammations, and Swellings: For skin irritations, try an ointment or cream prepared from marshmallow root and slippery elm (see recipe below), or make a poultice from the dried and ground root of marshmallow. Simply add a little water to make a paste from the powdered root and water, then apply it to the irritation. Both are equally effective, but the ointment seems to be easier to use and there is no need to worry about it falling off.

Skin Ulcers, Injuries, and Removing Foreign Objects: Marshmallow Root and Slippery Elm Ointment is highly effective in healing skin injuries of all kinds. It also helps in the extraction and healing of foreign objects below the skin such as splinters, and particles imbedded in scrapes and cuts.

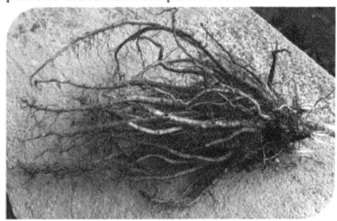

Marshmallow roots, by Victor M. Vicente Selvas, CCO

Urinary Tract Infections and Cystitis: Urinary tract infections and cystitis respond well to a decoction of Marshmallow root. It soothes irritated tissues and relaxes them, which helps with the pain and allows the decoction to work on the infection.

Recipes: Marshmallow Root and Slippery Elm Ointment: Ingredients: 100 g finely ground marshmallow root, 50 g lanolin, 50 g beeswax, 300 g soft paraffin wax, 100 g finely ground slippery elm bark. Heat the marshmallow root, lanolin, beeswax, and paraffin together in a double boiler or in a slow oven using the lowest setting. When cool enough to handle, but not yet set, stir in the slippery elm bark and pour it into a suitable container.

*You can also make this ointment without the slippery elm bark. However, the bark acts as a supplemental medicine and as a preservative to help the ointment keep longer.

Meadow Rue, *Thalictrum occidentale*

Meadow Rue, *Thalictrum occidentale*, is a perennial flowering plant. The herb is in the Ranunculaceae (Buttercup) Family. Despite its name meadow rue, Thalictrum is unrelated to the Rue Family, Rutaceae. Meadow rue is native to the western US, growing from Alaska and western Canada to California, Wyoming, and Colorado. It grows in moist and shady habitats such as meadows and forest understory.

Identification: Meadow rue grows to about 3 feet (0.9m) tall. The leaves of this herb are green in color, bipinnately compound and alternate. Leaves are divided into segments, often with three lobes, and grow on long petioles. The inflorescence is an upright or bent panicle of flowers, with male and female flowers growing on separate plants. The male flower is greenish white or purple, grows no petals, but instead has numerous dangling purple stamens. The female flower grows a cluster of up to 14 immature fruits with purple styles.

Edible Use: The only edible parts of meadow rue are the roots and young leaves. These roots have a bitter flavor and are rarely eaten. Instead they are used as

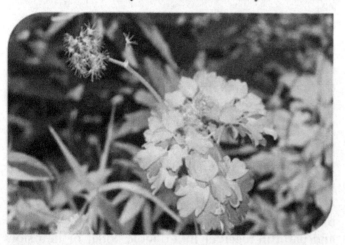
Meadow Rue, By Walter Siegmund, CC by SA 3.0

remedies to treat different ailments. Young leaves of meadow rue can be cooked and consumed as spinach.

Medicinal Use: Urinary Problems. A root decoction of meadow rue treats urinary problems.

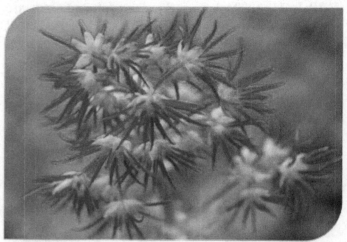
Female Flowers, photo by nordique, CC by SA 2.0

Reducing Fevers: Use a decoction from the roots or an infusion of the leaves to suppress fevers.

Cleans and Purifies the Body: Meadow rue is a general tonic that purifies the blood and cleanses the body.

Sores, Skin Infections, Piles: A poultice of meadow rue can be used to heal sores and skin infections. Crush and mash the root and leaves with a small amount of water for moisture. Apply the macerated herb to the area and cover it with a clean cloth to hold it in position.

Kill Lice and Other Vermin: Wash the hair and other body areas infected with lice, crabs, or other vermin with freshly made and warm Meadow Rue Decoction. Leave it on the skin for 30 minutes, then rinse it well. It should totally eradicate the problem. Follow up with a nit comb after killing lice.

Harvesting: Meadow rue can be harvested year-round. Uproot the plant then pluck off the young leaves and the roots. Wash the roots and the leaves and then dry them in a well-shaded place away from direct sunlight.

Meadow Rue Decoction: You'll need 1-ounce meadow rue roots and 1-pint (500ml) water. Crush or chop finely 1 ounce of meadow rue roots. Boil the root for 15 minutes or more to release the medicinal qualities into the water. Cool the decoction and strain it to remove the root fibers.

Milk Thistle, *Silybum marianum*

Milk thistle is known by many names, including blessed milk thistle, blessed thistle, cardus marianus, Mary thistle, Saint Mary's thistle, variegated thistle, Mediterranean milk thistle, and Scotch thistle. It grows in many places in North America and throughout the world. It prefers a warmer climate. It is in the Asteraceae /Compositae (Aster/Daisy) Family.

Identification: Milk thistle is an annual or biennial plant and grows from 2 to 6 feet (0.6 to 1.8meters) tall. The shiny green leaves are oblong or lance-like and can be either lobed or pinnate with distinctive white marbling. They are hairless with spiny margins and white veins. The stem is grooved and hollow in larger plants. Reddish-purple flowers appear from June to August. They are 1 to 5 inches (2.5 cm to 12.5 cm) across.

Edible Use: Eat milk thistle roots raw, boiled, parboiled, or roasted. The young shoots are harvested in the spring and boiled like spinach. Some people peel the bitter stems and soak them overnight before cooking them. Best to trim the leaves and stems to remove the spines before cooking or eating. You can eat the spiny bracts on the flower-head like a globe artichoke. Boil or steam them until tender. Milk Thistle is high in potassium nitrate and is not suitable for cattle or sheep.

Medicinal Use: Both the leaves and the seeds are used medicinally. The seeds can be eaten raw, and both the leaves and seeds can be used as a tincture, extract, or tea. You can grind the milk thistle seeds into a powder and put it into capsules for people who find the flavor disagreeable or need an easy way to take it. I make a tincture of milk thistle seeds and dandelion root for the liver. Silymarin, the most actively medicinal compound in milk thistle, is only found in the seeds.

Supports and Detoxifies the Liver: Milk thistle seeds are excellent at decreasing or even reversing liver damage caused by disease, environmental pollutions, chemotherapy, poisons, and drug or alcohol abuse. Milk thistle dramatically improves liver

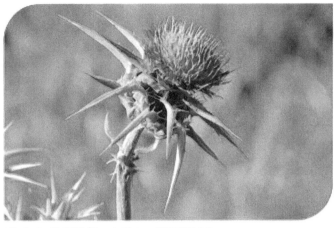

Photo by Fir0002/Flagstaffotos, GNU FDL 1.2,

regeneration in hepatitis, cirrhosis, fatty liver syndrome, and jaundice.

Prevents Gallstones and Kidney Stones: Milk thistle seeds support the endocrine and gastrointestinal systems and helps clean the blood. It works closely with the liver and other digestive organs to purify the body and reduce the risk of gallstones and kidney stones.

Helps Lower High Cholesterol: Milk thistle is a powerful anti-inflammatory with heart-healthy benefits, including lowering high cholesterol by cleaning the blood, decreasing inflammation, and preventing oxidative stress damage within the arteries. Milk thistle is effective in lowering total cholesterol, LDL cholesterol, and triglyceride levels in people with diabetes and heart disease.

Prevent or Control Diabetes: Milk thistle helps control the blood sugar and decreases blood sugar levels in insulin-resistant patients. For best results, use it regularly. The improved blood sugar control is due to the improved health of the liver and its function in releasing insulin and other hormones into the bloodstream.

Antidote for the Ingestion of Poisonous Mushrooms: Milk thistle seed's ability to protect the liver is so strong that it is even able to treat people poisoned by Amanita mushrooms, which destroy the liver. In fact, it is often the only treatment option for these patients and is given intravenously. Always be careful when harvesting and eating mushrooms. If you believe you've ingested poisonous mushrooms, seek medical help immediately.

Estrogen-Like Effects: Milk thistle leaves have some estrogen-like effects that stimulate menstruation and increase the flow of milk in breast-feeding mothers.

Cancer Treatment: Milk thistle seeds are sometimes used as a treatment for prostate, liver, and skin cancer, as silymarin has anticarcinogenic effects and protects the liver and kidneys during chemotherapy.

Acne: Milk thistle is high in anti-oxidants, anti-inflammatories, and flavonoids that reduce the inflammation of acne.

Harvesting: Always wear protective clothing and heavy gloves when harvesting milk thistle, as it is very irritating to the skin. Cut off young flower heads with scissors and young leaves from the stalk. Harvest milk thistle seeds by cutting off the seed-heads and placing them in a paper bag in a cool, dry spot. After the seeds dry, remove them from the seed head, one at a time, and brush away the debris. The cleaned seeds store best in a container with a tight lid.

Warning: Pregnant women should not use milk thistle. Women with estrogen-related conditions such as endometriosis, fibroids, and cancers of the ovaries, breast, or uterus should not use milk thistle. Do not use milk thistle if you are allergic to the Asteraceae/Compositae plant family.

Recipes. Milk Thistle Tea: Crush or grind 1 teaspoon of milk thistle seeds. Add one cup of boiling water and allow the tea to steep until lukewarm.

Milk Thistle Extract: Take 3/4 cup milk thistle seeds, 1 cup vodka or other alcohol, 80 proof or higher.

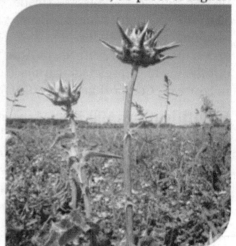

Grind, crush or blend 3/4 cups of milk thistle seeds. Place the crushed seeds into a sterile pint-sized (500ml) jar with a tight-fitting lid. Pour 1 cup of vodka over the seed, more if needed to cover the seeds. Stir well to mix the ingredients. Cap the jar tightly and place it in a cool, dark place for 6 to 8 weeks, shaking the jar daily. Add more alcohol, if needed, to keep the seeds covered with liquid. Strain the mixture and reserve the liquid. Discard the seed. Store your extract tightly covered in a cool, dark place.

To Use Milk Thistle Extract: This is a highly concentrated extract. Use three drops of Milk Thistle Extract up to three times daily. If this dosage is well tolerated, you can gradually increase the dose.

Mormon Tea, *Ephedra nevadensis*

Ephedra nevadensis belongs to the Ephedraceae Family. It is also known as Mormon Tea, Brigham Tea, Desert Tea and Nevada Ephedra. This herb is said to have gotten its name, Mormon tea, because of its use as a caffeine-free beverage by the Mormons. It is native to dry areas of southwestern North America and Central Mexico.

Identification: This desert shrub has jointed or fluted stems and scale-like leaves. Leaf scales of Mormon tea are in twos, 1 to 2 inches (2.5 cm to 5 cm) long, with sheathing to about the middle. The inflorescence of this plant is cone-like. The ovulate spikes of Mormon tea are distinctly stalked, and the seeds are usually

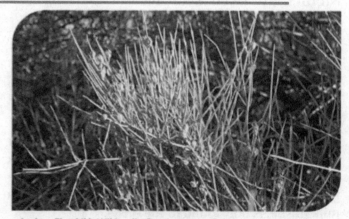

Andrey Zharkikh Wikipedia Commons, cc. 2.0

paired. This plant occurs naturally on flats and slopes in all the creosote bush deserts at mostly 1,000 to 4,000 feet (1219 meters) in elevation and sometimes it is found in desert grasslands up to 5,000 feet (1524 meters). The characteristic species that grow with this plant are Joshua tree, white bursage, black-brush, catclaw, burro-bush, black grama, bush muhly, and desert needle-grass.

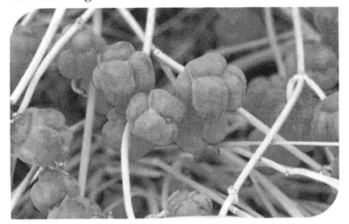

Ripe Female cones with seeds. Photo by Le.Loup.Gris, CC by SA 3.0

Edible Use: Both the fruit and seeds are edible. The fruit is sweet with a mild flavor, while the seed has a bitter taste and can be used cooked. It is sometimes roasted and ground to make bread. However, this plant is famous for its tea. Steep the green or dried twigs in boiling water until the tea turns an amber or pink color.

Medicinal Use: Mormon tea foliage is considered toxic but is used for medicinal purposes. It is a blood purifier, diuretic, fever-reducer, poultice, and tonic.

Urogenital Complaints: Use the stems for urogenital complaints including kidney problems, gonorrhea, and syphilis, if caught in its early stages.

Asthma and Respiratory Problems: Mormon tea and other members of the ephedra family are valuable for the treatment of asthma and respiratory system complaints. It does not cure asthma, but it opens the airways and relieves the symptoms of an attack. It is also useful for allergies and hay fever.

Heart Stimulant (Caution): Members of the ephedra family are known to contain ephedrine, which stimulates the heart and central nervous system. However, *Ephedra nevadensis* has little to none of the stimulant effects of ephedrine. However, drug potency varies from plant to plant, use it with care and do not use it on people with known arrhythmias or other problems where ephedrine is contraindicated.

Sores and Skin Infections: A poultice made from the powdered stems can be applied to sores for effective treatment.

Warning: Pregnant women and breastfeeding mothers should never use Mormon Tea.

Harvesting: Harvest the seeds of this plant by hand from native stands. On good years abundant collections of ephedra seeds can be obtained by flailing the fruiting branches over an open tray. Its stems can be harvested at any time of the year - dry them for future use.

Recipes: Mormon Tea Infusion. Break the stems into small pieces and wash them well. Add them to water and bring to a boil. Reduce the heat and simmer the twigs for 10 to 15 minutes. Once cooled, strain the liquid.

Mormon Tea: To make Mormon Tea, follow the instructions for Mormon Tea Infusion, then dilute the infusion with water until it is the strength you like. I dilute it to the color of tea. You can sweeten it with raw honey, if desired.

Mormon Tea Powder: Dry and powder the branches and twigs of the Mormon Tea Shrub. Moisten the powder to make a paste and use to make a poultice for sores and burns.

Motherwort, *Leonurus cardiaca*

Motherwort is a perennial member of the mint family that is often found at the edges of woodlands and in disturbed soils. It is widely distributed throughout North America and Europe and is sometimes considered invasive.

Identification: Motherwort is an upright bush that can grow to 6 1/2 feet tall (2m) and 3 feet (0.9m) or more wide. Motherwort leaves vary in size and shape along the stem. They are dark green on top and pale below. Lower leaves are deeply lobed with large teeth and can resemble maple or oak leaves.

They can reach five inches long and wide, and are hairy. Moving up the plant, the leaves become smaller with smaller lobes and teeth. At the top of the plant, leaves are usually small, narrow, and unlobed.

The stems are square, hairy, and branch only at the upper part of the plant.

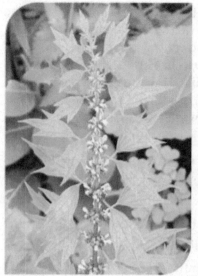

Photo by D. Gordon, Own Work, CC BY-SA 3.0

Hairy pale pink to lavender flowers grow in whorls alternating up the stem at the leaf nodes on the upper part of the plant. They bloom June through early September. The calyx remains on the plant through the winter, becoming brown and stiff when dry. Inside the lobes are 4 nutlets.

Edible Use: The flowers are edible and is used as a flavoring in pea soups, beer, or for making tea. The flavor is very bitter, so the leaves are rarely eaten.

Medicinal Use: Motherwort is best known for its benefits to the heart and for treating women's complaints. The leaves and flowers are the parts of the plant usually used for medicine.

Heart Health: Motherwort has a reputation for treating a wide variety of heart conditions. It is used to prevent calcification of the arteries, treating high cholesterol, hypertension, and other heart conditions.

Motherwort regulates the heart rate, treating rapid heartbeats and improves blood circulation in the body.

Prevents Strokes: This herb reduces the risk of blood clots forming in the body, thereby reducing the risk of strokes from blood clots.

Women's Health Issues (Birth, Delayed Menstruation, PMS): Expectant mothers use motherwort to reduce stress and tension at delivery time (do not take while pregnant). During delivery, it strengthens uterine contractions. It is believed that motherwort can also help the uterus recover after birth.

The herb is also effective at treating menstrual issues and regulating female hormones. It is an emmenagogue (stimulates menstrual flow) and thus helps with delayed menstruation. Herbalists use it to tone the uterus when menstruation is scant or to relieve cramps associated with delayed menstruation and PMS.

ADHD: Motherwort, along with Lemon Balm, Valerian, and Wild Oats, (Avena sativa), is often used to help people with ADHD.

Anxiety and Depression: Motherwort is believed to have a calming effect on the central nervous system and reduces stress, anxiety, worry, and panic attacks. It lifts the mood and reduces depression. For best results in reducing anxiety and depression, use motherwort regularly.

Hyperthyroidism: Motherwort relieves many of the symptoms of an over-active thyroid (hyperthyroidism). It regulates the metabolism, the nervous system, and relieves heart palpitations and anxiety caused by an over-active thyroid. It also helps increase the appetite and improves the overall thyroid health.

Insomnia and Sleep Problems: The calming effects of motherwort help improve sleep problems such as insomnia and restlessness.

Warning: Pregnant women should use the herb under the supervision of a medical professional. It can expedite labor and increase contractions.

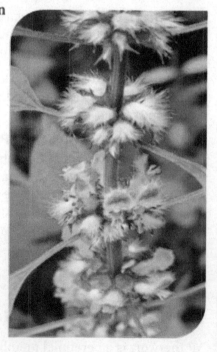

Consult a medical professional before taking the herb is you are taking heart medications or have heart problems.

Add the dried leaves to boiling water and allow it to steep for 10 minutes. Strain and enjoy. Sweeten the tea with honey or lemon if desired to improve the flavor.

Recipes. Motherwort Tea: 1 teaspoon of dried leaves, 1 cup of boiling water.

Motherwort Tincture: Motherwort leaves, stems, and flowers, roughly chopped, 80 proof vodka or similar drinking alcohol.

Glass jar, Sterilize a glass jar and tight-fitting lid. Fill the jar with chopped leaves, stems, and flowers to about 1/2 full. Fill the jar to within 1/4 (0.6cm) inch of the top, completely covering the herbs.

Cap the jar tightly and store it in a cool, dark place. Shake the jar once a day for six weeks. Check the alcohol levels regularly and add more alcohol as necessary to keep the jar full. Strain out the herbs and store the tincture in a sterile jar in a cool, dark place.

Mullein,
Verbascum thapsus

Mullein belongs to the Scrophulariaceae (Figwort/Snapdragon) family. It is most commonly known as great mullein or common mullein. Its other names include Flannel Plant, Aaron's rod, Hag Taper, Torches, and Velvet Plant.

Mullein is a widely distributed plant in North America and is exceedingly abundant as a naturalized weed in the eastern States. It grows in meadows, by roadsides, and on waste ground, especially on gravel, sand or chalky soil. This plant grows in a vast range of habitats but prefers disturbed ground.

Mullein is widely used for herbal remedies, with well-established emollient and astringent properties. This plant has also been used to make dyes and torches and is a lovely bush toilet paper.

Identification: Mullein is a velvety, soft, biennial plant. When in its second year, Mullein has an erect tall flowering spike that can reach nearly 8 feet (2.4 meters) in height. Its basal rosette, tall flowering stem, and velvety leaves make it easily recognizable.

Each mullein flower is about 3/4 inch (1.875 cm) across and consists of five pale petals, 5 hairy-green sepals, five stamens, and one pistil. In its first growth year, mullein leaves form a basal rosette. They have, very large, long, oval velvety, gray-green leaves that can grow up to 20 inches (50 cm) in length. In their second year, they send up a single tall flowering spike with alternately arranged leaves.

This plant produces small, ovoid capsules approximately 1/4 inch (0.625 cm) in length that contain many minute, brown seeds that are less than 0.04 inches (0.1 cm) in size.

Edible Use: The leaves and flowers are edible, although most people prefer them as a tea.

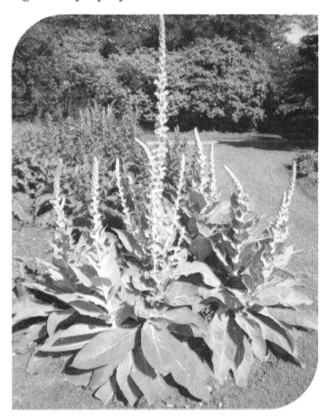

Medicinal Use: The leaves and the flowers of mullein are anti-inflammatory, antiseptic, antispasmodic, astringent, demulcent, diuretic, emollient, expectorant, anodyne (pain-killing) and vulnerary (wound-healing). I make an effective bronchitis tincture using Mullein, Lungwort Lichen and Yerba Santa for both symptomatic treatment and as a curative.

Bronchitis, Emphysema, Laryngitis, Tracheitis, Asthma, and Tuberculosis: Mullein is a commonly used herbal remedy. I value it for its efficacy in the treatment of chest complaints such as bronchitis, tuberculosis, and asthma. It reduces the

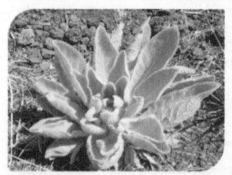

formation of mucus and stimulates the expulsion of phlegm. It is a specific treatment for tracheitis and bronchitis. For emphysema, try mullein infusion with some coltsfoot. The mixture of herbs acts well as an expectorant for emphysema patients and helps them breathe easier. It also relieves the coughing spasms and wheezing. People improve with long term use.

For asthma, mullein can also be inhaled. Mullein can be rolled into a rolling paper and smoked or, for children, the leaves can be burned and the smoke inhaled so as not to introduce them to smoking.

Skin Wounds, Snake Bite, Ulcers, Tumors, and Hemorrhoids: Externally, use a poultice prepared from mullein leaves to heal wounds, ulcers, tumors, and hemorrhoids. Mash the leaves, apply them directly to the skin, and cover them with a clean cloth. Mullein Infused Oil (recipe below) also works well on hemorrhoids. Mullein in a poultice form is drawing and may help draw out snake bite toxins if Plantain (*Plantago*) is not available – I would couple it with internal use. It also works to draw out splinters and the like.

Earaches and Ear Infections: I use an infusion prepared from its flowers infused in olive oil as earache drops. The flowers are strongly bactericidal. I usually mix mullein with garlic and yarrow infused in olive oil for ear infections. I put a few drops into the ear canal with a dropper and plug the ear with a cotton plug. I prefer to treat both ears, even if only one is affected, since the sinuses are connected. Do not use mullein (or any other oil in the ears) for punctured eardrums.

Sunburn, and Inflammatory Skin Conditions: Mullein is anti-inflammatory, which helps it to calm inflammatory skin conditions, especially those of the mucus membranes. For this purpose, I use a few drops of Mullein Infused Oil applied directly to the affected area. The oil also is anti-bacterial which helps

prevent infection and speed healing. I often pair St. John's Wort with mullein for sunburns.

Warts: Powdered mullein roots rubbed onto warts helps to kill the virus to the roots and remove the wart. Rub it in several times a day until the wart is completely gone and the skin is healed. The juice of the plant can also be used.

Cramps and Muscle Spasms: For cramping and muscle spasms, try an internal Mullein Infusion. For muscle spasms, Mullein Infused Oil can also be rubbed into the affected muscle.

Gastrointestinal Issues: Mullein Infusion made from the roots is very good for getting rid of intestinal worms and other gastrointestinal issues.

Harvesting: Mullein leaves are best harvested during the second year when the plant is growing a stalk. Harvest when the flowers are in bloom, usually between July and September. The flowers can be used either fresh or dried, although I prefer using them fresh when I can. To dry, bundle the leaves and hang them upside-down to dry.

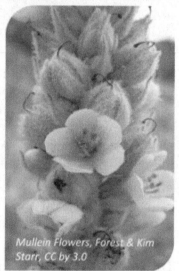

Mullein Flowers, Forest & Kim Starr, CC by 3.0

Warning: Do not use mullein if you are pregnant or breast feeding. In some people, it can cause skin irritations, stomach pain, and breathing difficulties. These are allergic reactions, so discontinue use if these symptoms occur.

Recipes. Mullein Infusion. Ingredients: 1/2 teaspoon powdered mullein root, and 1 cup water. Bring the water and powdered mullein root to a boil and reduce the heat to a simmer. Simmer for 10 minutes.

Mullein Infused Oil: Take 2 cups sweet almond oil or organic olive oil and 1 1/2 cups of mullein flowers, fresh or dried. Place 1 ½ cups of mullein flowers into a pint (500ml) jar with a tight-fitting lid. Pour the oil over the flowers and allow them to infuse for 3-4 weeks. Filter the oil and store it in a dark bottle in a cool, dry place.

Oregano, *Origanum vulgare*

There are many different varieties of oregano; all are medicinal but vary in the amounts of beneficial compounds. The most potent oregano is said to come from Greece and I find that plants grown in the summer heat seem to be more potent. It is in the *Lamiaceae* (Mint) Family.

Identification: You'll find oregano growing in most herb gardens and you may already use it in cooking.

If you are unfamiliar with it, look for bright-green, opposite oval leaves that are slightly hairy. It is a sprawling perennial plant that, like its relative mint, can take over an area. The plant grows close to the ground, reaching 8 to 32 inches (80 cm) tall. Each leaf is 1/2 to 1 1/2 inches long. The flowers are purple and tiny, growing on erect spikes above the leaves.

Edible Use: Oregano is used as a culinary herb to flavor many types of foods, especially in Mediterranean dishes.

Medicinal Use: For medicinal use, oregano can be used as an herb in food, used as a tea, as a tincture, or as an essential oil. The essential oil is very concentrated and should be diluted in a carrier oil before use. It is antiviral, antibacterial, and antifungal. Oregano is used internally to treat infections and externally to treat skin problems and fungal infections.

Boosts the Immune System and Antiviral: Oregano contains a wide range of antioxidants, anti-inflammatory, and anti-infectious properties that help the immune system heal the body faster. It contains vitamins A and C, as well as other compounds that are beneficial in boosting the immune system.

It helps relieve stresses on the body and stimulates the immune system to produce white blood cells, which defend the body against bacteria, viruses, fungi, and cancerous cells.

Yeast and Other Fungal Infections: Oregano oil is a powerful antibacterial, antiviral, and antifungal. It is also an anti-inflammatory, which helps in healing. It inhibits the growth of *Candida*, the yeast that most often causes yeast infections. Carvacrol and thymol are the main components that treat yeast infections and preventing them from spreading.

Use Oregano Tea or Tincture once or twice daily to treat internal yeast infections and for external use, use a tea wash or use well-diluted oregano oil. The diluted essential oil is effective against toenail fungus, athlete's foot, other fungal infections, and ringworm.

Skin Problems: Oregano contains antioxidants and anti-inflammatories that are beneficial to healing, reduce the signs of aging, heal blemishes, and reduce the appearance of scars. They neutralize the free radicals in the skin that cause wrinkles and age spots and they improve skin elasticity.

Cancer: In addition to the beneficial anti-inflammatory benefits and immune boosting effects of oregano for fighting cancer, the carvacrol in oregano has antitumor properties that slow the growth and reproduction of cancer cells and promotes cancer cell death.

Heart Healthy: Oregano Tea contains omega-3 fatty acids and helps improve cholesterol levels. It is also beneficial for the heart in other ways, helping prevent atherosclerosis, heart attacks, and stroke.

Stimulates Metabolism and Weight Loss: Oregano stimulates the metabolism causing the body to burn more calories. It can increase energy levels in some people and can help you lose weight.

Prevent Illness or Speed Recovery: When household members are sick, I often use Oregano Tea or Oil of Oregano to prevent the spread of the illness and to speed recovery of those who are ill. Best to use at the first sign of illness.

Bronchial Infections, Asthma, and Coughs: Add oregano oil to water and create a facial steam for loosening congestion and treating bronchial infections, asthma, and coughing. It relieves the inflammation in the airways.

Harvesting: You can usually find a starter plant at your local garden store. Harvest the leaves and stems before the plant blooms for best flavor. It is still potent after blooming, but the flavor is more bitter.

Warning: Do not take Oil of Oregano when pregnant. It is concentrated and has not been proven safe for pregnancy.

Recipes. Oregano Tea. I prefer to use fresh oregano leaves to make tea, though dried leaves can also be used. Dried leaves will lose the valuable oils and nutrients over time, so make sure your supply is fresh.

You need: 1 Tablespoon fresh oregano leaves or 1 teaspoon dried, 1 cup boiling water, raw honey or maple syrup to taste.

Crush or bruise the oregano leaves in the bottom of a cup or mug. Pour 1 cup of boiling water over the leaves and cover the cup to hold in the heat. Allow the tea to steep for 5 to 10 minutes. Add honey or maple syrup to sweeten the tea and make it palatable.

*To use as a wash, leave the tea unsweetened and allow it to cool before using it.

Oil of Oregano. The essential oil of oregano can be made by steam extraction. If you have the equipment for a steam extraction, it makes a stronger oil that must be diluted before use. See page 37 for instructions. The method below is easier, but it produces an oil that is less potent; no dilution is needed.

Oil of Oregano Infusion. Fresh oregano leaves and stems. Carrier oil such as organic olive oil, grapeseed oil, jojoba oil, or any other suitable oil. Gather several large handfuls of fresh oregano. Wash and air-dry. Chop the sprigs and leaves, bruising them to release the oils. Place the oregano into a clean glass jar, packed, but not overflowing. Heat the carrier oil on a very low heat and pour it over the oregano. Stir the oil gently to coat the oregano and release any air bubbles.

Cover the oil lightly (not sealed) and allow it to cool completely. Allow to steep for 1 week. Warm the oil again to release any moisture. Strain the oil, cover it tightly, and store it in a cool, dark place.

Oxeye Daisy, *Leucanthemum vulgare*

Also known as dog daisy, oxeye daisy is in the Daisy/Aster Family. It is often found in disturbed areas, fields, and roadsides throughout temperate North America, Europe, and Asia. It is an introduced species to North America.

Identification: Oxeye daisy is easily recognized by its white ray flowers with yellow center florets. Each erect plant grows 1 to 3 feet (0.3m to 0.9m) tall from well-developed shallow rhizomes. You'll often find them in groupings, spread by the reach of its rhizome underground. The leaves are long, lobed, irregular, alternate, and coarsely toothed. Leaves become progressively smaller as you go up the stem. Each stem holds one flower that blooms From May to October. It is often confused with Shasta Daisy (also edible), which is much taller.

Edible Use: The leaves, young shoots, flowers, and roots are edible. Young shoots and leaves are good chopped and added to salads. The flavor is strong, so I

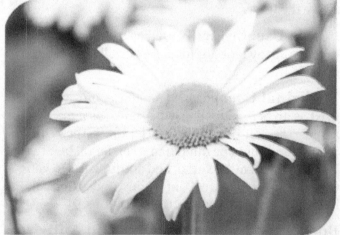

use them sparingly. The pungent flavor increases with age, so older leaves are best cooked, changing the water during cooking. They are good added to soups and stews. The roots can be eaten raw and are best in the spring.

Medicinal Use: The entire aerial part is medicinally active, but the flowers are most potent. The plant acts as an anti-inflammatory, antispasmodic, diuretic, and tonic. It induces sweating, relieves coughs, and heals wounds.

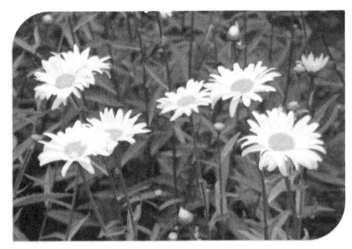

Chest Congestion and Coughing: Oxeye daisy is effective in relieving the coughing spasms of whooping cough and colds, and helping relieve congestion and mucous in the lungs. Try Oxeye Flower Tea or Tincture for this purpose.

Asthma: Oxeye daisy is an antispasmodic and helps relieve spasms in the airway, helping people with asthma breathe easier.

Tonic: Oxeye daisy is a mild tonic for the body, soothing irritation and inflammation in the body.

Wounds, Bruises, Rashes, Fungal Infections, and Other Skin Diseases: Oxeye daisy acts to soothe inflammation and irritations of the skin and is a good ingredient for lotions and salves. Used on the skin, it helps heal cuts, scrapes, bruises, insect bites and stings, and fungal infections. The tea or decoction can be used as a wash.

Eye Infections, Conjunctivitis: Boil the flowers in distilled water and strain through a fine mesh or coffee filter. Cool and use the sterile wash as an eye drop in the treatment of eye infections.

Detoxing, Diuretic Properties: Oxeye daisy is a mild diuretic and promotes sweating. It helps the body remove toxins through the urine and skin.

Insecticide and Flea Control: Dried flower heads, pounded or ground into a powder, are useful as a flea powder and as an insecticide.

Harvesting: Harvest the leaves, flowers, and stems while the plant is in bloom. Dry for future use.

Recipes. Oxeye Daisy Flower Tea: Boil oxeye daisy flowers, leaves, and stalks together, reduce heat and steep for 5 to 10 minutes. Strain and flavor with raw honey.

Peppermint, *Mentha piperita*

Peppermint is also called balm mint, curled mint, and lamb mint. The plant is easily recognized by its classic scent and flavor. Peppermint likes moist, rich soil and spreads quickly. It is indigenous to Europe but can be found worldwide. It is in the Lamiaceae (Mint) Family.

Identification: Peppermint is a perennial plant that grows from 1 to 3 feet (0.3m to 0,9m) tall. It has smooth, square stems and dark green opposite leaves with reddish veins.

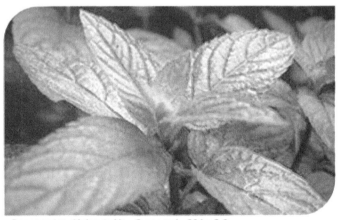

Peppermint, Aleksa Lukic · Own work, CC by 3.0

The leaves are 1 to 3 inches (2.5 cm to 7.5 cm) long and about half as wide. Leaves have coarsely toothed margins, a pointed tip, and are covered in short hairs. Purple flowers bloom from mid to late summer and are about 1/4 inch (0.6 cm) in length.

The flowers do not produce viable seeds and the plant spreads by underground roots and rooting stems.

Edible Use: Peppermint is edible and often used as a tea.

Medicinal Use: Gastroenteritis, Indigestion, Flatulence, Stomach, Intestinal, and Liver Problems: Peppermint leaves and tea are well known as a treatment for indigestion, excess gas, nausea, and other stomach upsets.

Peppermint oil stimulates the flow of bile in the body and aids digestion. It is useful for treating problems of the stomach, intestines, and liver. Peppermint oil also contains anti-bacterial and anti-viral components that treat the causes of gastroenteritis while also calming the symptoms.

Menstrual Cramping: Peppermint oil relaxes uterine muscle spasms and relieves menstrual cramping. Women with menstrual cramping can drink peppermint tea or take peppermint oil. The oil is very strong, so only a drop or two is needed.

Appetite Suppression and Stimulation: Peppermint temporarily inhibits hunger, but when the effect wears off the feeling of hunger returns more powerfully. It can be used as an appetite stimulate in this way, just be aware that it takes time to work. Good for children who are failing to thrive due to a lack of appetite.

Headaches and Migraines: The oil also relieves the spasms that cause some types of headaches. For this purpose, use a drop of distilled peppermint oil mixed into a tablespoon of a carrier oil like organic olive oil. Rub the oil onto the forehead or on the scalp over the affected area to relieve the headache. You may also use a peppermint oil infusion, though the distilled oil is stronger.

Diarrhea, Spastic Colon, Irritable Bowel Syndrome, and Crohn's Disease: Peppermint calms the stomach and intestinal tract, relaxes the muscles, and soothes the mucous membranes. It helps treat diarrhea, spastic colon, and irritable bowel syndrome by alleviating the spasms of the intestines and colon.

Itchy Skin: Peppermint oil slightly numbs the skin surface to relieve pain from insect stings, itchy skin, and mild skin irritations. It also has an anti-bacterial

component, and it works to bring an increased blood supply to the skin to speed up healing.

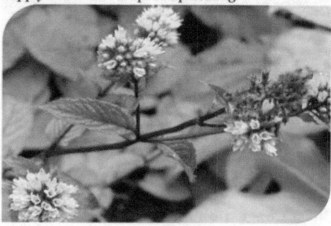
Peppermint Flowers, Sten Porse, CC by SA 3.0

Arthritis, Gout, Neuralgia, Sciatica: These same numbing qualities make it an effective treatment for muscle aches, joint pain, and nerve pain coming from near the surface. Massage the area with Infused Peppermint Oil (recipe below) to relieve the pain. It does not treat the underlying causes, but it gives quick relief from the pain.

Recipes. Peppermint Tea: 1 teaspoon peppermint leaves, 1 cup boiling water. Pour the boiling water over the peppermint leaves and allow the tea to steep for 10 to 15 minutes. Strain and drink.

Infused (Extracted) Peppermint Oil: 3/4 cup dried peppermint leaves, 1 cup organic olive oil. Combine the peppermint leaves and organic olive oil in a glass jar with a tight-fitting lid. Shake daily. Allow the oil and peppermint to steep in a dark cupboard for 4 to 6 weeks. Strain out the peppermint leaves and store the oil in a cool dark place for up to 1 year. Use as a topical relief for headaches, muscle cramps, or as a massage oil for muscle pain.

Plantain, *Plantago major*

Plantago major is a small perennial, often called a weed, and is not the banana-like fruit called plantain found in the grocery store. It is found growing wild in gardens, lawns, backyards, and along paths. It is in the Plantaginaceae Family.

Identification: The distinctive leaves have a ruffled texture. The leaves are oval or almost round and have a chunky footstalk. The leaves grow in a rosette at the base of the plant. Each leaf is 2 to 8 inches (5 cm to 20 cm) long. It has a wavy or smooth margin and five to nine parallel elastic veins. When you break the leaf in half and pull these elastic-like veins can easily be seen. The greenish-white flowers have purple stamens and grow on densely packed stems to a height of 6 to 18 inches (15 cm to 45 cm). The flowers are tiny and mostly eclipsed by the greenish-brown sepals and bracts. The flowering stalks rise high above the foliage. The plants produce many tiny, bitter-tasting seeds. *Plantago lanceolata*, narrow-leafed plantain, can be used like *P. major*.

Edible Use: The leaves and seeds are edible. I enjoy the leaves in a salad and gather them while they are still very young and tender and I love to strip the seeds and pop them in my mouth. As they age, they become tough and fibrous, but they can be cooked in soups and stews. The seeds are sometimes ground into a flour extender or substitute, but they are so tiny that it takes a lot of time and energy to gather enough to make it worthwhile.

Medicinal Use: The plantain herb has many medicinal qualities. It is anti-inflammatory, analgesic, antioxidant, demulcent, diuretic, expectorant, hepatoprotective, immune modulating, and a weak antibiotic.

Healing Wounds, Sores, Insect Bites, and Rashes: A poultice made from crushed plantain leaves is a good choice to promote healing in minor wounds, sores, and insect bites or stings. It will ward off infection, help stop bleeding, and reduce inflammation, taking away the sting or itch.

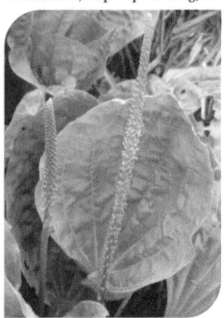

A spit poultice is easily made when you are bitten. Plantain has an excellent drawing effect, and can remove venom or a stinger. My kids know that if they get bitten or stung to chew some plantain and apply it for almost immediate relief. If a wound is infected, I combine plantain with an herb with more antibiotic action such as yarrow. To make a poultice, crush, chew, or bruise fresh plantain leaves and apply them directly to the affected skin. Cover the leaves with a gauze wrapping to hold it in place. Change the poultice as needed.

Snake Bite: For snakebite, use plantain both internally and externally. Apply a poultice of fresh plantain leaves directly to the bite to draw out the venom and

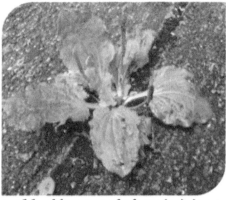

take 2 tablespoons of freshly pressed plantain juice or 1 teaspoon of Plantain Tincture. The tincture can also be used as a poultice if fresh leaves are not readily available. For snakebite, much depends on the kind of snake and the quick administration of remedies.

Cystitis, Diarrhea, Respiratory Tract Infections, Ulcers, and Colitis: The juice of common plantain leaves is beneficial for calming inflammation of the mucous membranes, including the membranes of the respiratory tract, digestive tract, and urinary tract.

Plantain for Autoimmune Diseases and Leaky Gut: For autoimmune conditions and other chronic diseases, try drinking Plantain Tea twice daily or take it in tincture form. The benefits build up over time. Just like Plantain works on your skin it also provides healing inside your gut. For Leaky Gut eat fresh leaves and drink it juiced or as a tea daily. Tincture is also effective but supplementing with fresh plantain or tea helps the plantain reach the gut lining for direct healing.

Toothache: The direct application of plantain on a toothache or dental infection is very effective in relieving swelling, infection, and pain. I like to combine it with the application of clove oil. Both can be soaked on cotton and packed into the infected area. Dried leaves can be used if fresh are not available.

Sore Throats and Swelling of the Gums: Add a tablespoon of pressed plantain juice to a half cup of water and use as a gargle at the first sign of a sore throat. It also reduces the inflammation in gum tissue.

Constipation, Intestinal Worms and Inflammatory Bowel Disease: Plantain seeds are excellent at relieving constipation and intestinal worms because of the fiber and mucilage released in the infusion. To relieve constipation, try drinking 1 cup of Plantain Seed Infusion (see recipe below) at bedtime. Be sure to consume the liquid and seeds for its full laxative effect.

Recipes. **Plantain Seed Infusion**: Take 1 teaspoon plantain seeds and 1 cup boiling water. Pour the boiling water over the seeds and allow it to steep while it cools. Drink the mucilage tea and the seeds. **Plantain Tincture**: You'll need plantain leaves, 80 proof vodka or other drinking alcohol and a glass jar with a tight-fitting lid. Fill the jar with fresh plantain leaves that have been chopped into small pieces or half a jar of dried plantain. Pour vodka over the leaves and fill

the jar, making sure all the leaves are covered. Cap the jar tightly. Let the tincture marinate for 6 to 8 weeks, shaking the jar occasionally. Pour the alcohol through a fine mesh sieve, cheesecloth, or a coffee filter to remove all of the herbs. Store the tincture in a cool, dark cupboard for up to 5 years. Dosage: 1/2 to 1 teaspoon. To infuse Plantain Oil substitute organic olive oil for the vodka and follow the same instructions.

Plantain Tea: Place 1 teaspoon dried plantain leaves or 1 tablespoon of fresh plantain leaves into a cup of boiling water. Let steep for 10 minutes. Strain out the leaves and drink.

Prickly Pear Cactus, *Opuntia ficus-indica*

The prickly pear cactus is in the Cactaceae (Cactus) Family. It is also known as Indian Fig, Barbary Fig, Cactus Pear, and Mission Cactus. It grows in the Southern United States and Mexico.

Identification: Prickly pear cactus grows up to 16 feet (4.8meters) tall with flat, rounded leaf pads that branch off. The flower and, later, the fruit, grow directly on the leaf pad. The entire cactus, including the fruit, is covered with two different kinds of spines. There are large, fixed spines that are easily seen and

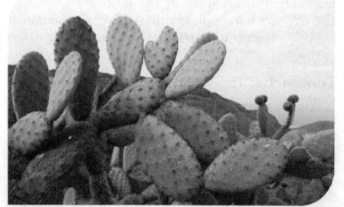

small, hair-like spines that are more difficult to see and easily detached. It is these smaller spines that can embed in your skin if you are not careful. The solitary flowers are large, bisexual, and yellow to orange in color. The fruit, called a tuna, is a berry covering numerous hard seeds. Prickly pear cacti are found in semi-arid and desert-like conditions and are easily cultivated in containers. They grow in bushy clusters.

Edible Use: Both the leaf pads and the fruit are edible. Peel them carefully before use (see Harvesting). Drink the juice of the tunas and use the pads in salads, tacos, stir-fries, and soups. The fruit is highly nutritious.

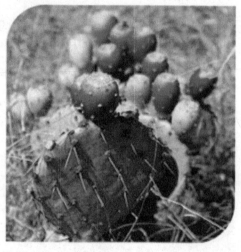

Medicinal Use: The anti-inflammatory effects of the prickly pear fruit are exceptional. Keep a supply of the dried fruit for travel, but the fresh juice is best. For maximum benefits, drink at least 2 ounces (60ml) of juice every day. There are no known health risks with long term use.

Arthritis and Joint Pain: Arthritic joint pain caused by inflammation is greatly helped by the regular consumption of prickly pear juice every day. Relief takes time (one to two months) and increases with use.

Snake Bite and as a Drawing Poultice: The prickly pear leaf is excellent as a drawing plant for toxins. Cut off the outer pad of the prickly pear leaf and mash the inner part and put on a snake bite as soon as possible.

Use it along with *Plantago* and *Echinacea*, if they are available.

Diabetes: Prickly pear cactus is beneficial to the pancreas, which is vital to insulin production. By restoring pancreal health, it helps balance blood sugar.

Heart Disease, Cholesterol and Circulation: The anti-inflammatory benefits assist in the reduction of plaques in the arteries and veins, reducing the chances of heart disease. Pickly pear juice also reduces cholesterol and enhances blood circulation to all parts of the body.

Muscle Soreness and Fatigue: The high vitamin and other nutrient levels combined with the health properties of prickly pear make it an excellent choice for the treatment of fatigue and muscle soreness caused by injury or over use.

All Inflammatory Diseases: The juice is indicated for all inflammatory diseases including skin diseases like psoriasis, eczema, and hives.

Harvesting: Harvesting prickly pear must be done carefully due to their small, hairy spines. Dress in thick long sleeves, long pants, boots, and gloves. I use tongs to pick the ripe fruit and leaves and place them carefully into a basket for processing.

After collection, I hold the fruit or leaf pad over a flame and burn the spines off completely, charring the skin. When they cool, I peel off the skin. Some people use sandpaper to remove the spines, but I prefer charring.

Prunella vulgaris, Self-Heal

Self-heal, *Prunella vulgaris*, is also known as wound root, woundwort, and heal-all. This low-growing plant attracts butterflies and bees. It belongs to the Lamiaceae (Mint) Family. I often find self-heal along roadsides and waste-places, but I prefer to harvest it from the edges of woodlands or grow my own in my garden.

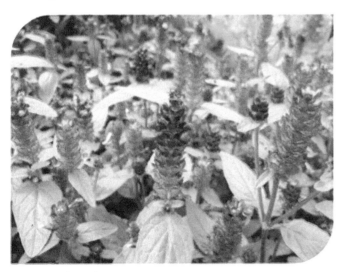

Identification: Self-heal is a perennial plant that grows 4 to 20 inches (10 cm to 50 cm) tall and produces small flowers from April to June and fruit from June to August. Each flower has a light purple upper lip and a whitish, fringed lower lip and a light green or reddish calyx that is hairy on the edges. Its fruit has 4 tiny seeds. Opposite leaves are lance-shaped and 1 to 3 inches (2.5 cm to 7.5 cm) long, growing on a single or a cluster of upright stems. The leaves have white hairs on the underside along the center vein. The leaf margins may be smooth or edged with blunt teeth. The root is a fibrous rhizome with a root crown and spreads through creeping stems that take root.

Edible Use: The young leaves and stems of self-heal are edible. They make a good addition to salads or can be boiled and eaten as a potherb. The aerial parts of the plant can be dried, powdered, and brewed into a cold tea.

Medicinal Use: The plant is nutritional and medicinal. It contains a number of vitamins, minerals, anti-inflammatories, and antioxidants. It is most famous for its use in treating cold sores, but it is also useful in treating a number of internal and external ailments. It is anti-inflammatory, antiviral, astringent, demulcent, hypotensive, immunomodulating, and vulnerary (healing). I usually use it as a complementary herb, using it in conjunction with other more powerful herbs. The entire plant is medicinal but the flowers, stems, and leaves are most commonly used.

Cold Sores and Genital Herpes: Self-heal treats both herpes simplex virus 1 (HSV-1 causes cold sores) and herpes simplex virus 2 (HSV-2 causes genital herpes). This herb has anti-viral properties. It prevents the virus from infecting host cells as well as reducing outbreaks.

Diabetes: Self-heal works to reduce insulin sensitivity in diabetes and pre-diabetes. It helps normalize blood sugar levels and prevents the development of diabetes related health conditions such as atherosclerosis.

Cancer: Research indicates that self-heal induces cell death in cancer cells. Cancerous tumor growth slows or stops with the use of the herb. Try the cold-water Self-Heal Tea or powdered herb in capsules for cancer alongside traditional treatments. Consult your doctor about your treatment.

Stimulates the Immune System: Regular use of self-heal herbs or Self-Heal Tea stimulates the immune system to help the body fight infections and even cancer. It also helps reduce swollen glands and helps clear toxins from the body.

Heals Wounds and Skin Infections: Self-heal's vulnerary, demulcent, and astringent properties stabilize wounded tissues and protects the skin. I use self-heal to treat cuts, burns, and skin wounds of all kinds. Internal wounds on the throat as well as mouth ulcers can be treated with self-heal. I treat surface skin problems, including infections and boils, with a poultice made from the herb and deeper inflammation with Self-Heal Tea.

Insect Bites and Stings, Rashes, and Poison Ivy: Juice from the stem of the plant, applied directly to the irritated tissue, is effective in calming the inflammation, burn, and itch of bites, stings, and rashes of all kinds. A poultice can be made from the plant for larger areas.

Viral Infections Including HIV: Self-heal's anti-viral properties are able to inhibit the growth of viruses in the body and prevent outbreaks. It prevents replication of the virus and helps stop the disease.

Respiratory Infections: Self-heal strengthens the immune system and helps the body fight off upper respiratory infections. It also treats sore throats and abscessed tonsils. Use Self-Heal Tea to treat respiratory infections and to soothe sore throats.

Allergies and Chronic Inflammation: Self-heal is an immunomodulator that regulates the immune system response and reduces chronic inflammation and seasonal allergies. It does not cure allergies but helps modulate the severity of the problem.

Kidney Problems and Hypertension: Self-heal strengthens the kidneys and promotes proper function. It also acts as a diuretic to help remove excess fluids from the body and lowers high blood pressure.

Heart Problems: Self-heal reduces high blood pressure and acts as a tonic for cardiovascular tissues. Regular use of Self-Heal Tea is said to strengthen the heart.

Liver Problems: Self-heal is useful in treating liver problems including hepatitis, jaundice, and a weak liver. It helps detoxify the liver and boosts its function. Use Self-Heal Tea regularly to treat liver problems.

Hemorrhage and Bleeding Caused by Extreme Menstruation: Self-heal stops internal bleeding, including excessive bleeding from menstruation. Take the herb as a tea or in capsule form for internal bleeding, as well as treating the underlying causes.

Digestive Problems, Colic, Crohn's Disease, Gastroenteritis, Ulcers, and Ulcerative Colitis: Self-heal helps to soothe the inflamed gastro-intestinal tissues, stop bleeding, heal ulcers and wounded tissues and fight bacteria, fungus, and viral infections, which contribute to the underlying causes of problems in the gastro-intestinal tract. It is also effective against the bacteria that cause ulcers and helps them heal. Try the herb in capsule form or a soothing Self-Heal Tea for treating digestive problems.

Self-heal also treats flatulence, diarrhea, gastritis, and intestinal parasites.

Hemorrhoids: Self-heal is useful topically to reduce the inflammation and irritation of hemorrhoids. Use a strong tea as a wash on the infected area or to make a compress for the area.

Harvesting: Harvest self-heal flowers when the blooms are open. Removing all flowers encourages the plant to flower again, but some flowers should be left at the end of the season to develop seeds. Dry the flowers and store in a cool, dry, and dark location until needed.

Warning: Self-heal should be used in moderation and is effective at low doses. Long-term use at high doses affects the internal organs, including the liver and kidneys. Self-heal can cause allergic reactions such as a skin rash, nausea, itching, and vomiting. Side effects can include dizziness, constipation, and weakness. The safety of self-heal in pregnancy has not been determined.

Recipes. Self-Heal Tea (Cold Water Infusion). 1-ounce dried self-heal herb, 1-quart (liter) of cold water, 1-quart (1 Liter) jar and lid. A cold infusion extracts some components that are destroyed by heat.

Tie the herbs up in muslin or cheese cloth and dampen the bag and herbs. Fill the jar with cold water and place the tied muslin bag into the water. Secure the string so that the herbs will float in the upper third of the water. Cold steep the herbs for one to two days or until the tea is to your taste. Remove the tea bag and store the remaining tea in the refrigerator until needed.

Pulsatilla, *Anemone pulsatilla* and *A. occidentalis*

This lovely flower is also known as anemone, Easter flower, Wild Crocus, Windflower, Pasqueflower, and Prairie Smoke. It is in the Ranunculaceae (Buttercup) Family.

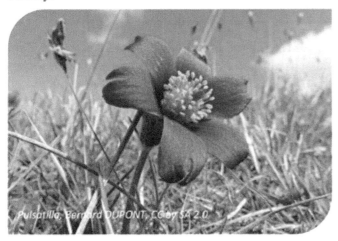

Pulsatilla, Bernard DUPONT, CC by SA 2.0

Identification: Pulsatilla is a perennial that grows 6 to 24 inches (15 cm to 60 cm) tall. The leaves are feathery, delicately divided, and covered with silky hairs. Each plant produces a single light purple or white flower with yellow stamens. The stamens produce feathery, hair-like seeds. These are one the first flowers to arrive in the spring, sometimes pushing through snow to make an appearance. The taproots run 3 feet (0.9m) or more into the ground. When the fruit head matures, the hair-like threads blow in the wind, giving the impression of smoke in the wind.

Medicinal Use: Use Pulsatilla leaves and flowers as either an infusion or a tincture. Pulsatilla must be used carefully and in small doses. In large amounts, it can be harmful or deadly. Avoid touching the fresh plant and only use dried flower heads and leaves in medicinal preparations. There are better options for most of the maladies below. Use with great care.

Skin Problems: For skin diseases, try a blended wash of Pulsatilla and Echinacea. Echinacea is an antibiotic and antiviral, and it stimulates the immune system. It works well with Pulsatilla to relieve skin problems related to inflammation and infection.

Menstrual Problems: Pulsatilla is very effective for menstrual pain, premenstrual tension, restarting menstruation, and menstrual cramping. It also relieves symptoms of menopause such as headaches, hot flashes, and moodiness.

Childbirth and Postpartum Depression: Pulsatilla stimulates the uterus and makes childbirth easier. It also has analgesic properties, which help with labor pain. It is also given after childbirth to relieve symptoms of depression. Either the tea or the tincture is used. Do not take earlier in pregnancy.

Headaches and Sleep Problems: Pulsatilla relaxes an overstimulated nervous system and treats headaches and insomnia. It calms the body and spirit allowing people to sleep soundly when taken in small doses. Note that Lemon Balm also accomplishes this without the dosing risks of Pulsatilla.

Mental Disorders and Panic Attacks: Because of its actions on the nerves, Pulsatilla is useful

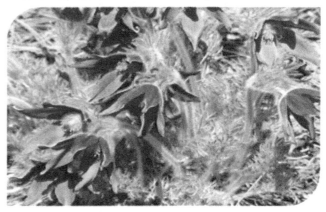

for treating nervous conditions including: hyperactivity, senile dementia, panic, and schizophrenia.

Eye and Ear Problems: Pulsatilla possesses many properties that are beneficial to the eyes and ears. The tea is useful in treating cataracts, conjunctivitis, glaucoma, and tics. The tea is also used to treat earaches, hearing loss and inflammations of the ear.

Heart Health: Pulsatilla is beneficial to the heart in numerous ways. It is used to cure thickening of the heart muscle and clear venous congestion. It relieves inflammation in the circulatory system and helps restore normal function. However, it should not be used for people with slow heart rates (bradycardia).

Drug Withdrawal: Pulsatilla is useful to help with withdrawal from sedatives, hypnotic drugs, anticonvulsants, and muscle relaxants. Be careful to give only the prescribed dosages of Pulsatilla Infusion or tincture.

Harvesting: Pick Pulsatilla flowering stalks and leaves when the plant is in full bloom, usually in the early spring near Easter.

Warning: Pulsatilla should never be used internally for pregnant women.

Given in large doses, Pulsatilla can be harmful and may cause coma, seizures, asphyxiation, and death. It can also cause a slowing of the heart rate. Wear gloves when harvesting Pulsatilla flower heads. Use only the dried flower heads and dried leaves in herbal preparations. The fresh herb is an irritant.

Recipes. Pulsatilla and Echinacea Tea: 1/2 teaspoon dried Pulsatilla flowers, 1 teaspoon dried Echinacea root and leaves and 1 cup boiling water. Pour the boiling water over the herbs and allow them to steep for 10 minutes. Strain and drink.

Purslane,
Portulaca oleracea

Purslane is another of those backyard weeds that is under appreciated. While it is usually considered a weed, it is an excellent groundcover, vegetable, and medicine. I love to eat it in a salad. It has a salty, sour flavor that adds variety with its taste and texture. It is in the Portulacaceae (Purslane) Family and is also called common purslane, pigweed, little hogweed, verdolaga, or red root.

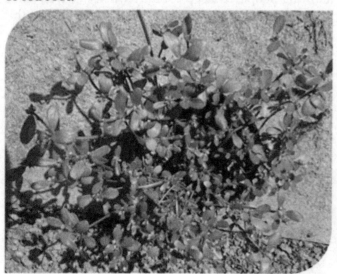

Purslane by JeffSKleinman, CC SA 4.0

Identification: *Portulaca oleracea* is a succulent that sprawls along the ground. It grows about 6 inches tall (15 cm) in a wide mat. Purslane stems are smooth and reddish or pink. The deep green thick leaves grow in groups at the stem joints and ends. Leaves can be alternate or opposite. Small yellow flowers, growing in clusters of two or three, appear in late summer and open for a few hours on sunny mornings.

Each flower has five parts and is up to 1/4 inch (0.6 cm) wide. Seeds form in tiny pods that open when the seeds are mature. The plant has a deep taproot and fibrous secondary roots. These help it survive poor soils and periods of drought. It prefers a sunny spot with dry soil.

Edible Use: Purslane has a sour, salty flavor and can be a little bitter when leaves are mature. Purslane leaves, stems, and flowers are edible raw, cooked, and pickled. When cooked like spinach, it can be a bit slimy.

Cooked purslane does not shrink as much as most greens, so a small patch can provide vegetables for an entire family. The leaves can be pickled to provide purslane during the winter months. Seeds can be collected and ground into a flour.

Medicinal Use. Uterine Bleeding: Purslane seeds are used for abnormal uterine bleeding. It helps decrease the volume and the duration of bleeding.

Asthma and Bronchial Complaints: People who eat purslane in vegetable portions or take purslane extract show improvement in overall pulmonary function.

Purslane helps with shortness of breath and opens bronchial tubes to increase oxygen reaching the lungs. For asthma attacks and other bronchial conditions, try a Purslane & Mullein Mix (recipe below). Therapeutic effects of purslane for respiratory diseases are indicated in ancient Iranian medical books. The bronchodilatory effect of the extract of *Portulaca oleracea* in the airways of asthmatic patients was examined. The results of the study showed that purslane has a relatively potent but transient bronchodilatory effect on asthmatic airways.

Diabetes: Purslane seeds or their extracts are effective in improving serum insulin levels and reduce triglycerides with long-term, daily use. People report lower blood sugar readings and better management.

Fungal Infections: Purslane has antifungal properties against the most common causes of athlete's foot, jock itch, and ringworm. Apply purslane extract to affected areas several times a day, until the infection is gone.

Lower Cholesterol: Purslane naturally lowers cholesterol due it its high pectin content. Take 1

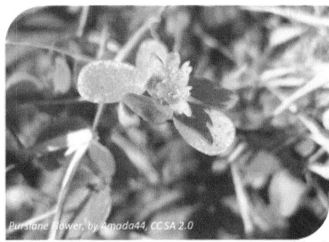
Purslane Flower, by Amada44, CC SA 2.0

teaspoon of purslane tincture or 2 teaspoons of fresh purslane juice daily.

Cancer: Gastric Carcinoma and Colon Adenoma. Purslane leaves and seeds have been shown to be an anti-cancer medicine for certain cancers. It also has a high Omega 3 and gamma-linoleic acid content. It is an excellent anti-oxidant.

Warning: Purslane is considered safe to eat in large portions without any side effects.

Recipes. Purslane & Mullein Mixture for Asthma: 3 droppers of Purslane tincture, 1 1/2 droppers Mullein tincture, 1/4 cup water. Add the Purslane and Mullein tinctures to the water. Note that when measuring with a dropper, the dropper will not fill up; this is fine. Drink the mixture in part or in full as needed.

Red Clover, *Trifolium pretense*

Red clover is a member of the Fabaceae (Pea) Family. I often find it growing along roadsides and fields. It is a biennial or short-lived perennial that grows to 18 inches (45 cm) tall.

Identification: The plant grows from a long, deep taproot and slender, hairy, hollow stems. The leaves are alternate, divided into three leaflets, and green with a pale crescent in the outer half of the leaf. Leaflets are 1/2 to 1 1/5 inches (0.25 cm to 3.125 cm) long and 1/2-inch (0.25 cm) wide and fine-toothed with prominent "V" marks. Pink to red flowers appear in rounded heads from May to September.

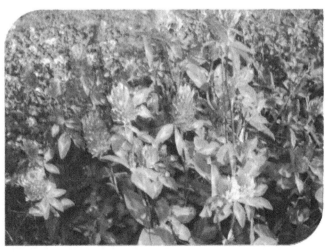
By Sanja565658 - Own work, CC BY-SA 3.0

Edible Use: I eat the leaves and young flowering heads both raw and cooked. The flowers make a sweet herbal tea and the ground seed pods and flowers can be used as a flour substitute. The taproot is edible when cooked.

Medicinal Use. How to Use Red Clover: Red clover can be taken as a dried herb, tincture, or as a tea made from the blossoms.

Relieves Symptoms of Menopause: Because of its phytoestrogen isoflavone content, red clover flowers work as a natural alternative to hormone replacement for women. It relieves symptoms of menopause, including reducing the frequency of hot flashes and night sweats. I usually pair it with Black Cohash for menopause symptom relief.

Osteoporosis: By acting as a natural hormone replacement, red clover may slow bone loss and even boost bone density in pre- and peri-menopausal women.

Cardiovascular Health: Red clover helps protect against heart disease by increasing HDL (good) cholesterol in pre- and post-menopausal women. It also has blood-thinning properties, which improve blood flow and prevent clotting.

Skin Conditions Including Eczema, Psoriasis, and Other Skin Irritations: Red clover flower tea, supported with yellow dock and nettles, is an excellent internal remedy for skin irritations. Use an external poultice made from chopped red clover flower and water applied directly to skin lesions.

Harvesting: Harvest red clover from fields, away from heavy pollution areas such as roadsides. Unlike most herbs, red clover needs to be harvested in the early morning while there is still some dew present on the flower.

Pick the blossoms one to two weeks after blooming. Snip the blossom head off and leave the rest of the plant alone.

Use the blossoms fresh or place them on a drying rack in a warm dark, ventilated, and dry place. Turn them frequently until the blossoms are dried through. Store the dried herb in a cool, dry, and dark place. When harvesting young leaves, try to get them before the plant flowers.

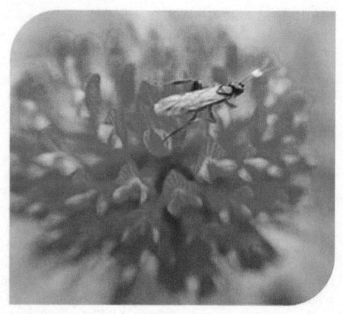

Guttorm Raknes, Own work, CC by SA 4.0

Use them cooked as a green, in soups, and salads. The leaves can also be dried and powdered for use as a flavoring on foods. They tend to be more bitter after the flowers appear.

Warning: In general, red clover is very safe, with few side effects, except for occasional gas. The anticoagulant effect and hormonal effects may be undesirable for some people.

Due to its hormonal activity, don't use red clover for women with a history of endometriosis, breast cancer, uterine cancer, fibroids, or other estrogen-sensitive conditions.

Red clover contains coumarin derivatives and must be used with caution in individuals taking anticoagulation therapy. Also, do not take red clover before surgery or childbirth. It can inhibit blood clotting and healing.

Recipes. Red Clover Tea (hot): Red clover blossoms, fresh or dried, and 1 cup boiling water. Steep three fresh red clover blossoms or 2 to 3 teaspoons of dried flowers in 1 cup boiling water.

Allow the tea to steep while cooling for 15 minutes. Drink warm or allow to cool for external use. Drink up to three times daily for maximum benefits.

Red Clover Tea (Cold): Add one-half cup of red clover blossoms to a quart (a liter) of water and allow it to steep in the refrigerator for 24 hours.

Rosemary, *Rosmarinus officinalis*

I love the scent and flavor of rosemary. I use it mainly to flavor potatoes and lamb and as a medicinal herb. It grows easily in a garden. It is in the Lamiaceae (Mint) Family.

Identification: Rosemary, is a woody herb with fragrant needle-like leaves and a fibrous root system. It is an evergreen shrub that can withstand extreme droughts. Most bushes are upright reaching 5 feet (1.5m) tall, but some can develop into trailing plants. The leaves look like hemlock needles. They are green on the top and white on the underside, with both sides covered with short, dense, wooly hair. White, pink, purple, or blue flowers appear in the spring and in the summer in cooler climates and year-round in warmer climates.

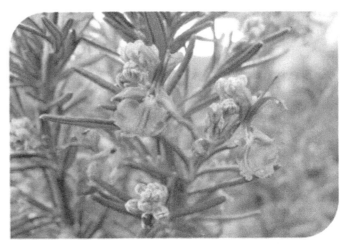
Rosemary in bloom, Margalob, CC by SA 4.0

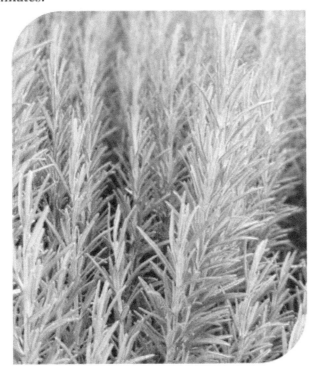

Edible Use: Rosemary is often used in cooking. The leaves and the flower petals are edible and nutritious.

Medicinal Use: Rosemary contains caffeic acid, carnosic acid, carnosol, and rosemarinic acid, anti-inflammatories, and anti-oxidants.

Stimulates Digestion: The stimulant properties of rosemary bring circulation to the digestive organs and help relieve digestive problems, especially indigestion. You may use rosemary in your food and/or use a tincture or infused oil before a large meal.

Improves Concentration and Memory, Neuroprotective: Rosemary is known as a brain tonic. It seems to improve concentration and memory. It stimulates the circulatory system, bringing more oxygen to the brain. It is used for elderly dementia patients. It also has a neuroprotective effect due to the carnosic acid found in rosemary.

Circulatory Problems and Headaches: Rosemary is a mild stimulant, well-known for increasing circulation. Use it for problems with the cardiovascular system, poor circulation, and low blood pressure. These same stimulant properties make it a good choice for alleviating headaches, especially migraines. Rosemary has a mild analgesic effect, but the main relief comes from opening up the blood flow to the brain.

Inflammation, Colitis, Arthritis: The analgesic properties and anti-inflammatory properties help reduce the pain and swelling of joints inflamed from arthritis. People report that it helps their pain and swelling but does not completely alleviate it, so it usually used in combination with other herbs. It also reduces gut inflammation.

Antifungal: Rosemary is a good antifungal and I often add rosemary essential oil to an external antifungal salve.

Antibacterial: *Pseudomonas* and Staph: Rosemary essential oil inhibits the bacterium *Pseudomonas*. It also works to kill *Staphylococcus*, as does oregano oil.

Anti-cancer and Hepatoprotective: Rosemary has been researched for a variety of cancers and it has many properties, such as caffeic acid, carnosic acid, carnosol, and rosemarinic acid that help fight cancer. It also protects the liver.

Hair Loss: Rosemary essential oil has been shown to be as effective as the prescription hair growth drug Minoxidil. Apply in a carrier oil on the scalp (I prefer coconut oil) and keep using long-term.

Halitosis: Rosemary makes an extremely effective mouthwash. It can get rid of bad breath very quickly. Gargle and rinse with Rosemary Mouthwash every morning and night, more often if needed. A mouthwash recipe is below.

Recipes. Rosemary Mouthwash: Bring 2 cups of water to a boil and remove it from the heat. Steep 1 heaping tablespoon of dried rosemary flowers and/or leaves in the water for 30 minutes. Store the mouthwash tightly covered in the refrigerator for up to 3 days.

Queen Anne's Lace, *Daucus carota*

Queen Anne's lace is often used as an ornamental. It is also known as wild carrot because of its carrot scent and because it is a member of the Apiaceae (Carrot) Family. Be careful with identification as there are look-alikes, like the deadly hemlock plant. My favorite story to tell them apart is about Queen Anne sewing a piece of lace. She pricked her finger and a single drop of blood fell into the center of the flowers, symbolizing the single red or purple flower in the center of each umbel. The presence of this blood colored flower is a positive identification for Queen Anne's Lace. As a rule, if you are unsure don't pick it.

Identification: Queen Anne's Lace grows to 1 to 4 feet (0.3m to 1.2m) tall. The flower stems are green, hairy, and may have long red stripes. They are thin and have a thin hollow space in the center. Clusters of flowers, called umbels, are arranged in a tight pattern

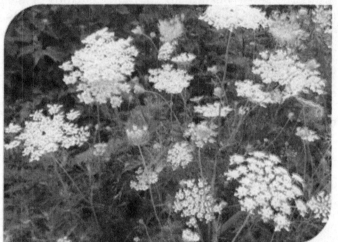

gathered into a larger umbrella shaped cluster. The umbels are flat across the top and 3 to 4 inches (7.25 cm to 10 cm) wide. Blooms may be pink in bud and white when in full bloom. In the center there is a single reddish or purple flower. Seeing this red or purple flower is a definitive marker for Queen Anne's lace, but not all varieties have the color.

When the flowers die, Queen Anne's lace flowers curl into a bird's nest shape as they dry. Leaves on Queen Anne's lace are lance-shaped serrated leaflets. Each leaf is 2 to 4 inches (5 cm to 10 cm) in length and slightly hairy on the underside. The plant has a single thin taproot that is shaped like a carrot.

Edible Use: The thin taproot from Queen Anne's lace is edible cooked, however it quickly becomes very fibrous and woody as growth progresses. For eating purposes, only young roots are tender enough to cook and eat. The flowers are edible and are good battered and fried. The first-year leaves are edible in small portions. Caution is necessary when handling or eating the plant because of its close resemblance to poison hemlock. Make sure of your identification before consuming any herb! Remember: Queen Anne has hairy legs.

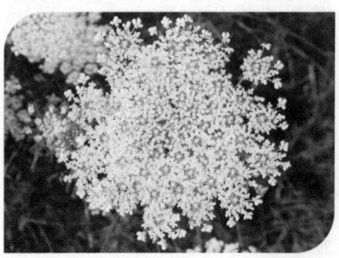

Queen Anne's Lace, Jrosenberry1, CC 4.0

Gallstones, Kidney Stones, Chronic Kidney Problems, Bladder Problems, and Gout: Queen Anne's lace seeds and roots are used for treating gall bladder problems and kidney problems. It acts to remove excess water from the body and reduce inflammation.

Colic, Upset Stomach, and Flatulence: The soothing and diuretic properties of the root are helpful for treating stomach and intestinal upsets.

Skin Problems: For itchy dermatitis, a poultice made from the grated root helps relieve an itchy rash.

The seed oil is also good for soothing and lubricating the skin. It is also anti-inflammatory.

Birth Control and Conception: Queen Anne's Lace seeds have been used to prepare the womb for pregnancy when used before ovulation. If taken after ovulation or as an emergency contraceptive seeds should be used for 3 days. Use with care. Do not use during pregnancy!

Warning: Do not use while pregnant or nursing. There are a lot of poisonous look-alikes so be careful with proper identification.

Sage, *Salvia officinalis*

There are many different varieties of sage, and many of them have medicinal properties. Here we are discussing common sage. I try to use it in cooking so that I get the beneficial compounds often. It is in the Lamiaceae (Mint) Family and is easy to cultivate in the garden.

Identification: Common sage grows to approximately 2 feet (0.6m) tall and wide. It flowers in late spring or summer, producing lavender, purple, pink or white flowers. Leaves are oblong, approximately 2 1/2 inches (3.75 cm) long and 1 inch (2.5 cm) wide. The leaves are grey-green colored and wrinkled on the top, while the underside is white and covered in short, soft hairs.

Edible Use: Sage is commonly used as a cooking herb.

Medicinal Use: Sage is an antiseptic, antimicrobial, anti-mutagenic, antibacterial, helps stop neuropathic pain, improves memory, lowers blood glucose levels, and alleviated menopause symptoms. It is an excellent all-around herb.

Digestion Aid: Sage help in the digestion of rich, fatty meats, which perhaps is why it is used so often in sausage recipes. Its stimulant properties work to move fats through the digestive system efficiently and prevent indigestion.

Balances Hormones for Men and Women: Sage is effective in balancing

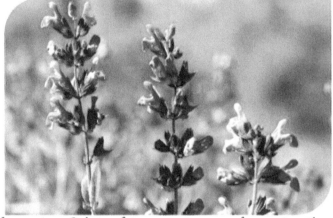

hormones. It is used to promote normal menstruation and to treat menopausal symptoms such as hot flashes, night sweats, headaches, and mental fog. It is also useful in treating premature ejaculation in men.

Sore Throats: The most effective remedy is a gargle, but many people object to the flavor. Thus we have added a recipe below for a better-tasting throat spray that is almost as effective. Both remedies contain several herbs that fight infection and calm the inflammation of a sore throat.

Speed Healing in Wounds: For slow-healing wounds, make a compress by soaking a cotton pad in sage infusion. Apply the cotton pad to the wound and hold in place with tape or a clean piece of cloth or gauze. The sage infusion relieves the pain almost immediately, fights infection, and brings more blood to the area to speed healing.

Hair Growth: Sage essential oil improves blood circulation to the scalp and roots of the hair. This encourages thick hair growth and is often paired with rosemary essential oil.

Warning: Sage can significantly reduce the amount of milk produced in nursing mothers. Avoid its use when breastfeeding.

Recipes. Sage Throat Spray: 3 tablespoons dried or fresh sage leaves, 3/4 cup boiling water, 1/4 cup Echinacea Extract, 1 tablespoon raw honey. Pour the boiling water over the sage leaves and allow it to steep for 30 minutes. Strain out the leaves. Add the Echinacea extract and raw honey. Store in a bottle with

a spray top, preferably with a fine mist. Spray in the back of the throat as often as needed.

Sage Gargle for a Sore Throat: This gargle doesn't taste great, but it works! 1 tablespoon dried sage leaves, 1 cup boiling water, 1 teaspoon goldenseal root powder, 5 drops Cayenne Infusion, 1/2 cup apple cider vinegar, with live culture.

Pour the boiling water over the dried sage and allow it to steep for 45 minutes. Strain out the leaves and add the goldenseal root powder, cayenne infusion, and vinegar. Gargle with this mixture every hour for as long as you can stand it. Spit out the gargle.

Sheep Sorrel, *Rumex acetosella*

Sheep sorrel is one of the most useful medicinal herbs, and yet many people pull them out or spray them to rid their yard or field of it. Sheep sorrel is also known as red sorrel, narrow-leafed dock, spinach dock, sour weed, and field sorrel. It is a member of the Polygonaceae (Buckwheat) Family. The plant grows as a common perennial in most areas.

Identification: Sheep sorrel has small green leaves shaped like arrowheads and deeply ridged, upright red stems that are branched at the top. The plant grows to 18 inches (45 cm) tall at most. It grows from an aggressively spreading rhizome.

Sheep sorrel blooms from March to November and are either all male or all female. Yellowish-green male flowers or maroon colored female flowers grow on a tall, upright stem. The maroon female flowers develop into red achenes. It is one of the first species to appear when an area has been disturbed.

Edible Use: Sheep sorrel is edible raw as a salad green or as a garnish. The flavor is tart and lemony. It can be used as a curdling agent during the cheese-making process and can be cooked like spinach.

Livestock will eat the plant, but it is not very nutritious and can cause problems if too much is consumed because of its high concentration of oxalates.

Medicinal Use: Use sheep sorrel leaves as a juice, tea, and powder or capsules.

Detoxification: Sheep sorrel is useful for detoxification. It has a diuretic effect and flushes the body when ample water is consumed. It also has laxative effects. For detoxification, use freshly juiced leaves or Sheep Sorrel Tea, though the tea and powder are less effective than the fresh juice.

Gastro-Intestinal Problems, Kidney, and Urinary Tract Diseases, Cysts, Swellings, and Skin Cancers: For tumors, swellings, cysts, and cancers close to the skin surface, use a leaf poultice. Apply the macerated leaf poultice directly over the affected area several times daily until the problem is resolved.

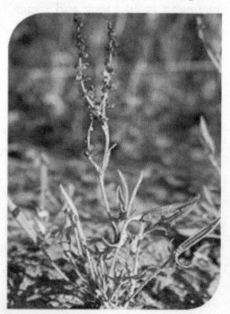

Henripekka Kallio, CC by SA 3.0, Female flowers Sheep Sorrel,

Intestinal Parasites and Worms: Use the tea internally to kill and flush worms and intestinal parasites out of the system. One cup of tea, taken twice daily for two weeks does the job.

Colds, Flu, and Sinusitis: Sheep sorrel is an excellent treatment for reducing the inflammation and pain that accompanies colds, flu, and sinusitis. The tannins help reduce the production of mucus and its anti-microbial action helps kill bacterial infections. Use sheep sorrel as soon as the illness begins to reduce the severity of the disease.

Warning: Because of its high oxalate content, people with kidney stones, arthritis, or hyperacidity should not use sheep sorrel.

Sheep Sorrel Tea: You'll need 1 teaspoon dried sheep sorrel leaves and 1 cup water.

Bring the water to a boil and pour over the dried sheep sorrel leaves. Cover and let the tea steep for 5 to 10 minutes. Drink warm.

Skullcap, *Scutellaria lateriflora*

Skullcap is also called blue skullcap, side-flowering skullcap, Quaker bonnet, hoodwort, mad dog skullcap, helmet flower, and blue pimpernel. It is a calming herb, useful for anxiety and nervous disorders of all kinds. It is in the Lamiaceae (Mint) Family. It likes moist areas throughout much of North America, where it is native, and is cultivated in much of Europe. North American skullcaps can be used interchangeably for medicine. Note that they are used differently than Chinese Skullcap (S. baicalensis), another useful herb.

Identification: The plant has smooth, square erect stems that reach 1 to 4 feet (0.3m to 1.2m) tall. The stems are leafy and branched, with oblong, opposite toothed leaves. Each leaf is 1 to 3 inches (2.5 cm to 7.5 cm) long, with smaller leaves at the top of the stems. The 2-lobed helmeted flowers are blue-violet to whitish. Each flower is about 1 inch (2.5 cm) long and grows in short spike-like racemes or singularly in the axils of the upper leaves. The flowers are tubular and the upper hooded lip gives it its name of "skullcap". Each flower produces 4 nut-like fruits. It blooms from July through September.

Medicinal Use: Skullcap is usually used as a hot tea or tincture, but some people prefer to use powdered skullcap in capsule form. Tinctures should be made with fresh herbs for optimal potency. Skullcap seems to act upon benzodiazepine GABA receptors in the brain. GABA is a neurotransmitter that helps prevent overstimulation of the nervous system. If it gets too low you can have seizures, epilepsy, anxiety, depression, insomnia and more.

American skullcap interacts with these GABA receptors, binding to the benzodiazepine site, as does Valerian and California Poppy, both in this book. The leaves, stems, and flowers are used medicinally,

though many people only use the leaves. The plant is rich in vitamins, minerals, and tannins. The plant is relaxing and acts as a natural tranquilizer and sleep aid. It is similar to valerian root in properties and activity.

Anxiety, Tension, Depression, and Insomnia: Skullcap relaxes the nervous system, reduces stress, and relieves anxiety. It reduces body tension and allows the body to relax into sleep. It calms people who are overly nervous, hysterical, or unable to relax.

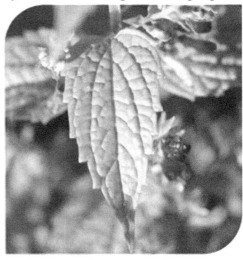

Its antioxidant properties help with oxidative stress, which is associated with depression and anxiety disorders, and it binds to benzodiazepine GABA receptors in the brain.

Millspaugh, C.F(1854-1923) Commons Wikipedia

Antioxidant and Neuroprotective: Skullcap is an excellent antioxidant and functions as a neuroprotective for diseases such as Alzheimer's and Parkinson's.

Muscle Spasms and Tension, Muscle, Seizures, Twitches, Calms the Nervous System: Skullcap is an antispasmodic. It eases muscle twitches, spasms, and seizures by relaxing the muscles, relieving involuntary muscle movements, and calming the nervous system.

Tension Headaches and Perhaps Migraines: People taking skullcap report that it helps relieve tension headaches. It may also help migraines.

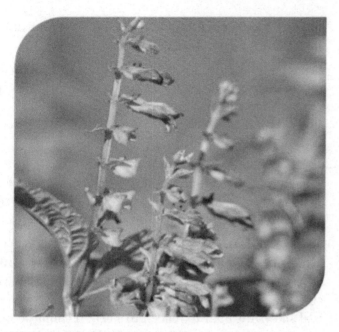

tremors, relaxing the mind, and relieving anxiety and depression.

Exhaustion and Depression: Skullcap is calming and allows the body and mind to rest. This is essential in treating exhaustion and depression. With good sleep and a calm mind, the body is able to put itself back in order and heal mentally and physically.

Harvesting: Wait to harvest skullcap until the plant is in full bloom. Remove stems, leaves, and flowers by pruning off the top of the plant, leaving approximately 3 to 4 inches (7.5 cm to 10 cm) to regrow. The herb is most potent when freshly harvested, but can be used dried.

Warning: Do not take skullcap while pregnant or breastfeeding. Safety is unknown. Use skullcap sparingly in small doses. Large doses may be harmful or could cause liver damage.

Drug Withdrawal, Smoking Withdrawal, Alcohol Withdrawal: Skullcap helps with withdrawal from drugs, especially benzodiazepines like Valium and Xanax. It also assists with withdrawal from alcohol and smoking by calming the body, relieving

Recipes. Skullcap Tea: 1 Tablespoon fresh skullcap leaves or 1 teaspoon dried, 1 cup boiling water, raw honey or Maple Syrup, if desired. Crush the herbs and place them in a tea ball. Pour 1 cup of boiling water over the herbs and steep for 5 to 10 minutes. Remove the teaball and sweeten the tea, if desired.

St. John's Wort, *Hypericum perforatum*

St. John's Wort, also called Klamath Weed, is recognized as an invasive weed in most parts of North America. It gets its name from its uncanny ability to bloom on June 24, the birthday of St. John the Baptist. It is in the Hypericaceae (St. John's Wort) Family.

Identification: St. John's Wort is an herbaceous perennial with creeping rhizomes. The stems are erect and grow up to 3 feet (0.9m) tall. The stems branch in the upper section and produce narrow, yellow-green leaves that are less than 1 inch (2.5 cm) long. The leaves have tiny oil glands that look like small windows when the plant is held to the light. Bright yellow flowers, measuring 1 inch (2.5 cm) across, appear on the upper branches from late spring to mid-summer. The flowers have five petals with pointed sepals. The sepals have noticeable black dots. The large stamens are grouped into three bundles and the flower buds have a red resin when squeezed. The plant is widespread. It likes dry soil and sunny locations.

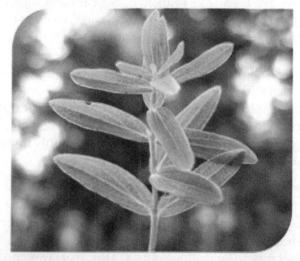

Medicinal Use: The flowers and leaves are used for medicine. They are best used fresh if available.

Depression, Anxiety, SAD and OCD: St John's Wort is most commonly used for treating depression, restlessness, anxiety, and insomnia without adverse effects. People with bipolar disorder should not take it, as it seems to increase the risk of mania. It should also not be taken by people already on an SSRI medication. It is very effective for SAD (Seasonal Affective Disorder) and OCD and is often paired with Lemon Balm.

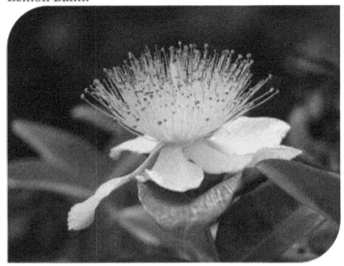

Menopause, PMS and Menstrual Cramping: St John's Wort reduces the symptoms of hormonal imbalances in menopause including depression and fatigue. It helps balance the hormones and stimulates the organs, increasing the tone of the uterus. It is also beneficial for relieving cramping, bloating, and mood symptoms of PMS.

Opiate Withdrawal and Quitting Smoking: St John's Wort helps with the symptoms of mild opiate withdrawal and aids people trying to quit smoking. It calms the nervous system and alleviates the physical symptoms of withdrawal from opiate-based drugs and helps relieve anxiety and depression for people quitting smoking. Use an internal St John's Wort Tincture for this.

Cuts, Bruises, Burns, Sunburns, and Other Injuries: Extracted St John's Oil is an excellent antiseptic and anti-viral and contains tannins that facilitate healing. Apply topically to heal burns, sunburns, injuries, wounds, and infections.

Neuralgia, Bell's Palsy and Nerve Pain: Nerve pain and neuralgia benefit from topically applied oil and internal tincture or tea. You can also use it for sharp and convulsive trigeminal neuralgia and sciatica. Apply the oil or salve on the affected areas 3x/day.

Muscle Pains: For back pain, muscle pain, and general body aches, use St John's Wort Oil or salve. It is useful taken internally and when massaged externally into the muscles.

Peptic Ulcers, Gastric Problems: St John's Wort attacks ulcers and gastric problems by calming the digestive organs and by attacking the bacteria and viruses that are causing the problem. It is effective against infective digestive problems such as gastroenteritis, dysentery, and diarrhea.

Hemorrhoids: The oil of St John's Wort is almost a miracle cure for hemorrhoids. It effectively reduces the inflammation, relieves the pain, and speeds the healing process. Use the recipe below and apply topical to the affected area 3x/day.

Epstein Barr Virus, Shingles, Hepatitis and Herpes Virus: The healing properties of hypericin, found in the petals and stems of St. John's Wort, may work as an anti-viral. It can also be applied externally for herpes and shingles outbreaks.

Removing Fluids and Toxins: The diuretic properties of St John's wort help to remove fluids from the body and flush away toxins through urination.

Bedwetting in Childhood: Giving 5 to 10 drops of St John's wort tincture in the late afternoon can help children with bedwetting problems. Flushing the excess fluids out of the system before bedtime helps prevent the buildup of fluids in the bladder.

Arthritis and Gout: St John's Wort reduces inflammation and pain, relieving the symptoms of these joint diseases. For best results, use it daily as the benefits increase over time as the inflamed joints heal.

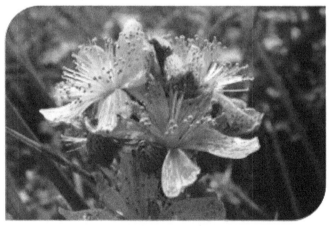

Chest Colds, Congestion, and Respiratory Disease: In addition to the anti-inflammatory and anti-microbial benefits of St John's wort, it is also an effective expectorant that helps clear chest congestion and phlegm. It speeds healing of infections and common coughs and colds. It is also used against influenza.

Warning: St John's Wort interacts with a lot of modern medicines. It should not be taken by people already on an SSRI medication and may cause sun sensitivity to very fair-skinned people. It may interact with Warfarin, Digitoxin, and HIV medications. Do not take for 2 weeks prior to surgery. Check with your physician before using.

Recipes. St John's Wort Tincture: Ingredients: St John's Wort flowers and leaves, 80 proof grain alcohol or vodka, a clean jar with a tight-fitting lid.

Loosely pack the flowers and leaves into the glass jar, filling it to the top. Add the alcohol to the jar, covering the flowers and leaves. Cap the jar tightly. Label. Add more alcohol as needed to replace evaporation. Shake the jar daily and allow it to steep for 4 to 6 weeks. Strain the herbs out. Cap the jar and keep it in a cool, dark cupboard. Take the tincture for a prolonged period as needed to cure chronic conditions.

St John's Wort Infused Oil: Four ounces(112g) of fresh St. John's Wort flowers and 2 cups organic olive oil. Mix the herbs and olive oil in a double boiler and place them over very low heat.

Steep the oil and herbs for 2 to 3 hours, keeping the oil at a low simmer. Strain the oil and remove the herbs. Store your infused oil in a cool, dark cupboard.

*St John's wort oil works well on its own, however, it can be even more healing when mixed with other herbs.

Stinging Nettle, *Urtica dioica*

I love stinging nettle, though I know many who don't due to its sting. It is nutritious, medicinal, and makes beautiful fiber. I even have a nettle shirt! Dock usually grows near it and can be used to take away the sting. It is in the Lamiaceae (Mint) Family.

Identification: Stinging nettle is a perennial, growing from 3 to 8 feet (0.9m to 2.4m) tall. It is dioecious and herbaceous, dying back in the winter.

The leaves are mostly oval or occasionally heart-shaped. The soft, green leaves are 1 to 4 inches (2.5 cm to 10 cm) long and are arranged oppositely on a square erect stem. The leaves have a serrated margin and cordate base. Both the leaves and stems are very hairy with non-stinging hairs and many stinging hairs. Numerous flowers appear June to September in dense inflorescences. They are greenish or brownish, growing in branched clusters. Male and female flowers grow on separate plants or branches. Stinging nettle is widely distributed, especially where the average annual rainfall is high. I find it in places with moist soil.

Edible Use: The leaves are edible. Stinging nettles have a flavor similar to mild spinach when cooked. I eat them raw by folding over the leaves but most people blanch them in water to remove the sting before cooking and eating. Only eat stinging nettle leaves before the flowers appear. Beyond that time, they can cause internal irritation, especially of the urinary tract. The seeds are also edible. Dried nettle leaves and flowers make a nice herbal tea.

Medicinal Use: Nettle can be taken as a tea or tincture and is my number one go to for allergies.

Allergies (including Hay Fever): Stinging nettle tincture is my first recommendation for allergies as it usually completely alleviates the problem. I often recommend coupling it with local raw honey. It is an excellent anti-inflammatory.

Arthritis, Gout Pain, and Inflammation: Stinging nettle treats arthritis, gout, and other inflammatory conditions. It suppresses inflammation, flushes toxins from the body, and helps reduce the pain of these conditions.

It is used in Germany as a treatment for Rheumatoid Arthritis and is thought to inhibit the cascade of inflammation. Externally, a compress made by soaking a cotton pad in nettle tincture and placing it over the painful joint is helpful. Stinging an area can also help restore and repair joint injuries and reestablish nerve communication. I have used it successfully to treat shoulder injuries.

Eczema and Skin Inflammations: Both the internal tincture and infusion of stinging nettle are useful for treating eczema and other skin inflammations.

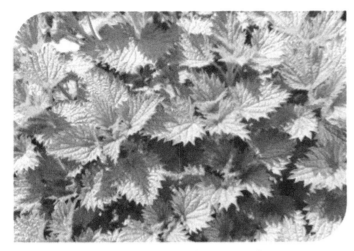

Burns, Insect Bites, and Wounds: Use a double strength Nettle Infusion as a wash to treat burned skin, sunburns, insect bites, wounds, and other skin irritations. Stinging nettle has combudoron, which has been shown to help with burn treatment. Make the Nettle Infusion recipe using 2 tablespoons of dried or fresh nettle leaves. Use the cooled liquid to wash and treat these conditions, allowing it to dry on the skin.

Menstrual Problems: Women with heavy uterine bleeding and other menstrual problems benefit from stinging nettle.

Sprains, Cramps, Tendonitis, and Sciatica: Muscle cramping, injuries and nerve pain benefit from the application of a compress made by soaking a cotton pad in Nettle Tincture and applying it over the affected area. Fasten it in place for best results.

Stimulates Blood Flow: Stinging nettle stimulates the circulatory system and blood flow. To stimulate blood flow and improve circulation, use a Nettle Infusion or Tea. It can also be used externally as the sting brings healing and blood flow to the area.

Anemia, Cardiac Insufficiency, Swellings, Enlarged Spleen and as a Whole-Body Tonic: For serious conditions such as these, use fresh nettle juice prepared by soaking and blending the whole fresh plant.

Hair Rinse: Use Nettle Tea as a hair rinse to increase shine. Couple it with Horsetail and Rosemary for maximum results.

Recipes. **Nettle Infusion**: You will need 1 tablespoon dried and crushed nettle leaves and 1 cup boiling water. Pour the boiling water over the nettle leaves and allow it to steep for 10 to 15 minutes. Strain and drink twice daily.

Nettle Tincture. Ingredients: stinging nettle leaves, fresh or crushed and dried (fresh is best), 80 proof vodka or other drinking alcohol of same strength, a glass jar with a tight-fitting lid.

Fill the jar with fresh nettle leaves that have been sliced into thin pieces and crushed. Pour vodka over the leaves and fill the jar, making sure all the leaves are covered. Cap the jar tightly. Label it. Let the tincture infuse for 4 to 6 weeks, shaking the jar daily. Add more alcohol if needed to keep the jar full. Pour the alcohol through a fine mesh sieve or a coffee filter to remove all of the herbs. Store the tincture in a cool, dark cupboard for up to 5 years. Dosage: 1/2 to 1 teaspoon, twice daily.

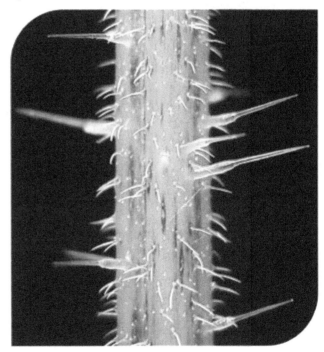

Stinging nettle, Frank Vincentz - Own work, CC by SA 3.0

Sweet Grass, *Hierochloe odorata* or *Anthoxanthum nitens*

This fragrant grass is also known as vanilla grass and holy grass, and is considered a sacred plant and is used ceremonially by many. It is native to Northern Eurasia and much of North America. It is in the Poaceae (Grass) Family. It is also used for weaving.

Identification: Sweet grass is a perennial grass that is hardy in extreme cold. The fragrant grass blades are not stiff and after it reaches about 8 inches (20 cm) tall it leans over and grows horizontally until the end of summer, reaching about 3 feet (0.9m) in length. Its blades are shiny and smooth and, if you look under the soil, you can see a broad smooth leaf base. The undersides are light in color.

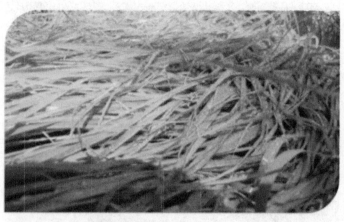
Sweet Grass, Kodemizer, CC by SA 3.0

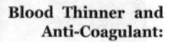

Medicinal Use: The leaves are used for medicine. It contains coumarin, an anti-coagulant.

Blood Thinner and Anti-Coagulant: Sweet grass contains coumarin, which transforms in the body into an anti-coagulant. Coumarin also gives sweet grass its sweet smell. Do not use on people with bleeding issues. Use carefully; excess can be toxic.

Common Colds, Bronchial Congestion: Inhale the smoke from burning sweet grass to treat common colds and congestion or drink the leaves as a tea for colds.

Insect Repellent: Two compounds found in sweet grass, phytol and coumarin, work as well as DEET in repelling mosquitoes.

Sore Throats, Coughs, Fever, Venereal Disease: Sweet grass leaf tea is used to treat sore throats, coughs, and fevers as well as venereal diseases. Use internally with care.

Harvesting: Harvest sweet grass throughout the summer, cutting it above the ground in the amounts needed. Best used fresh throughout the summer and dry a supply at the end of summer for winter use.

Warning: Be careful with internal use. Large doses can be carcinogenic and toxic. Use with great care.

Sweet Marjoram, *Origanum majorana*

Sweet marjoram, also called pot marjoram, is a tender perennial herb with a piney-citrus flavor. It is related to oregano and has some similar uses and a milder flavor. The plant is widely cultivated in herb gardens and can be found growing wild where it has escaped cultivation. I grow it in my garden for easy access. It is in the Lamiaceae (Mint) Family.

Identification: Sweet marjoram has smooth narrow opposite leaves approximately 1/5 to 3/5 inches long that are oval in shape with a slight point. The margin is smooth and the base is tapered. The leaf has numerous hairs that give it a smooth, velvety texture. The grey-green leaves are aromatic and flavorful. It grows to a height of 10 to 24 inches (60 cm) on several thin boughs. The stems are square and purple. The plant produces delicate white or pink blossoms on spikes at the end of the branches during late summer and early autumn.

Edible Use: The leaves, flowers, and stems are all edible.

Medicinal Use: The leaves of this herb have many medicinal uses and can be taken in food, or the distilled oil can be used.

Digestive and Respiratory Tonic: Sweet marjoram is an effective tonic for the digestive and respiratory tracts. It is an excellent treatment for problems related to these areas.

Menstrual Aid: The herb is capable of inducing menstruation and should never be used in significant amounts by pregnant women. Used in medicinal quantities, it calms the uterus and relieves pain and cramping. It balances the hormones and relieves the symptoms of menopause and pre-menstrual syndrome. It helps bring on menstruation when delayed.

Polycystic Ovarian Syndrome: People with PCOS and its related fertility problems may find relief with sweet marjoram. By balancing the hormones, it is able to relieve the symptoms of this disease and is said to help women to conceive.

Promotes Breast Milk Production: Nursing mothers report an increase in breast milk production when eating marjoram daily.

Diabetes: People with type II diabetes can add sweet marjoram and rosemary to their daily diet. The combination aids the use of insulin in the body and improves blood sugar management.

Muscle Spasms, Tension Headaches, and Over-Used Muscles: Marjoram essential oil has a calming effect on muscles and tension headaches. Some people say that simply breathing in the oil is enough to relieve a tension headache. Two or three drops added to a vaporizer or bath water is enough. It is also very effective for relieving muscle spasms and pain when diluted and used as a massage oil.

Lowers Blood Pressure: Sweet marjoram essential oil lowers blood pressure through breathing in the scent of marjoram essential oil. The relaxation of the body and release of stress helps lower the blood pressure naturally.

How to Use Marjoram Medicinally: As little as one tablespoon of dried marjoram, sprinkled on food, taken in capsules or used as a tea is enough to derive health benefits. For fresh herbs, add a quarter cup of chopped marjoram on your salads or other foods. Both the fresh and dried herb are beneficial.

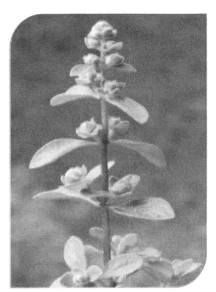

Warning: Do not use in high doses if pregnant, as it can bring on menstruation.

Thorn Apple,
Datura stramonium

Thorn Apple is a member of the Solanaceae (Nightshade) Family and must be used with care. Like other family members, it can be highly beneficial for medicinal purposes when used carefully in very small doses, and it can be deadly when used improperly.

It is also called jimsonweed, moon flower, and devil's snare. It grows wild across the warmer parts of the United States. It is often found in farm yards and along roadsides.

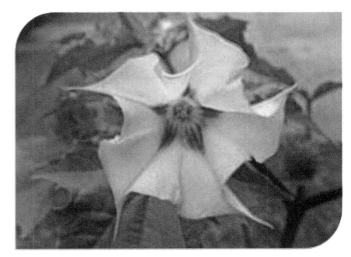

Identification: These 2 to 5-foot-tall annual bushes are foul-smelling, freely branching, and erect. The plant grows from a long, thick, and fibrous root. Stems are stout, leafy, smooth, and pale yellow-green. They form many forks and branches, with a leaf and flower at each fork. Leaves are 3 to 8 inches (7.5 cm to 20 cm) long, soft, irregularly undulated and toothed. The surface is smooth, with a darker green upper surface and a light green underside.

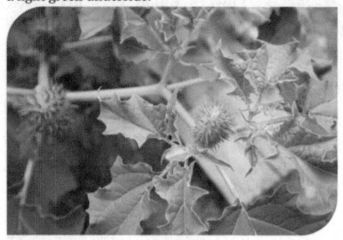

White, creamy, or violet trumpet-shaped flowers appear throughout the summer. Flowers are approximately 2 to 4 inches (5 cm to 10 cm) long on short stems growing from the branch forks or the leaf axils. The calyx is swollen at the base, long and tubular and surrounded with five sharp teeth. The corolla is only partially open and has prominent ribs. The flowers open at night.

Seeds are egg-shaped capsules, approximately 1 to 3 inches (2.5 cm to 7.5 cm) in diameter and either bald or covered with spines. When mature, it splits into four chambers, each containing many small black seeds.

Medicinal Use: The leaves and seeds are used in medicine. Traditionally the leaves are smoked. Today, some people use a Thorn Apple Seed Salve for external use and have discontinued using the herb as a smoke or extract because of its toxic effects. It is similar to Belladonna (deadly nightshade) in its constituents.

Asthma: Thorn apple leaves have long been smoked in cigarette or pipe form, mixed with tobacco, for the treatment of asthma.

I do not recommend this method since over-consumption causes delirium and hallucinations and even death. Mullein is a much better choice.

Burns, Wounds, Boils, and Skin Inflammations: A salve made with thorn apple seeds reduces inflammations in burns and other skin wounds and inflammations. The seeds have pain-relieving and narcotic properties.

Whooping Cough and Other Coughs: The narcotic and anti-spasmatic properties of thorn apple seeds are potent and useful in severe cases of whooping cough and muscle spasms.

Muscle Spasms and Parkinson's Disease: The tremors of Parkinson's disease and other muscle spasms respond to the anti-spasmatic properties of the seed extract. Start with the minimum dose and increase it only if necessary.

Warning: The plant contains dangerous levels of toxins and has a significant risk of overdose when used without medical supervision. Toxicity can also vary from plant to plant and with the maturity of the plant, so a safe dose one year might be toxic the next year as the plant matures. Use thorn apple only under the supervision of a highly skilled medical professional.

Recipes. Thorn Apple Seed Extract: 1/4 teaspoon thorn apple seeds, 1/4 cup 80 proof alcohol. Mix the alcohol and crushed seeds together in a small bottle and cover tightly. Allow the mixture to steep for 2 to 4 weeks. Strain out the seeds and store the extract in a cool, dark place for up to 3 years. Keep out of reach of children and mark it clearly as a poison.

Dosing: It is impossible to accurately recommend a dosage since the strength of seeds from each individual plant varies. Start with 1 drop and increase the dosage only as needed to get the desired effects. Watch carefully for symptoms of toxicity. Use only under medical supervision.

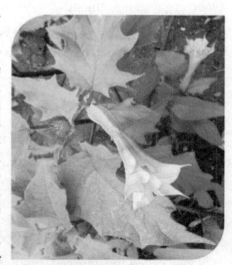

Thorn Apple, Skäpperöd, CC by SA 3.0

Thorn Apple Oil or Salve (For external use only): You will need 1/4 teaspoon thorn apple seeds, 1/2 cup coconut oil or olive oil (coconut oil is preferred if you want a solid salve). Place the coconut oil and crushed thorn apple seeds together in a small glass jar. Place the jar and its contents into a pot of barely simmering water. Keep the water level so that the jar stands upright and does not float. Maintain a very low simmer for 2 hours. Turn off the heat and allow the oil to cool. Strain the seeds out of the oil and discard them. Use the cooled oil as a rub or salve on painful joints.

Thyme, *Thymus vulgaris*

Thymus vulgaris is the same evergreen herb that we use for cooking. It is a member of the Lamiaceae (Mint) Family. This fragrant plant grows in hot, sunny locations.

Identification: Thyme is a perennial shrub with square stems growing from a thin woody base. It grows 6 to 12 inches (15 cm to 30 cm) tall. The leaves are small, light-green, and slightly curved. Small purple or white flowers appear in the summer.

Edible Use: I use it as a cooking herb for its intense flavor and as an herbal tea.

Medicinal Use: The Romans used thyme to purify their rooms and to flavor cheese and liqueurs. It has been placed under pillows to aid sleep and prevent nightmares. Thyme is an antiseptic, anti-viral, anti-parasitic, and anti-fungal. I prefer to use fresh thyme whenever possible. However, I also dry thyme sprigs for future use.

Sore Throat, Coughs, and Bronchitis: The anti-bacterial components of thyme are valuable in combatting bronchitis and coughs. Infuse the whole herb in water and use it for gargling and as a weak thyme tea.

Mouthwash, Dental Cavities and Gum Disease: Weak thyme tea is a valuable mouthwash. It has

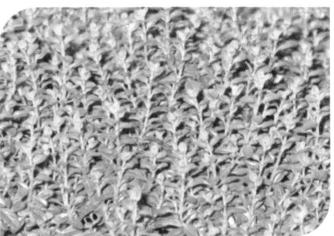

antiseptic properties, which help prevent cavities and treat gingivitis.

Acne: Try Thyme Tincture for treating acne. Dab a drop of thyme tincture onto blemishes once or twice daily. It dries up acne and kills the bacteria that cause them.

Boosts the Immune System: The many vitamins, minerals, and antioxidants in thyme give the immune system a boost. Also, thyme encourages white blood cell formation and increases the body's resistance to bacteria and viruses. Thyme based formulas, Thyme Tea, and Thyme essential oil are all good formulas for boosting the immune system.

Digestive Upsets and Worms: Thyme is effective against digestive problems caused by bacteria and viruses, including stomach flu and diarrhea. It is also used for intestinal problems, including worms.

Seizures and Antispasmodic: Thyme has antispasmodic properties and prevents and treats epileptic seizures in some people. Oil of Thyme or Thyme Tincture are the best products to use for this purpose.

Lice, Scabies, and Crabs: The anti-parasitic properties of thyme oil make it a good treatment for lice, scabies, and crabs. Add a few drops of Oil of Thyme to olive oil or coconut oil and coat the affected area. Cover the coated areas and leave on for 1 hour, then wash away. Follow up with nit removal and repeat as needed.

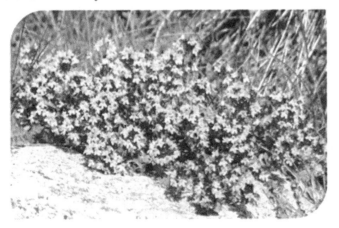

Skin Inflammations: Try a Thyme Leaf Poultice for skin inflammations and sores. Mash the leaves into a paste, place it on the skin over the affected areas and cover it with a clean cloth.

Warts: Mix one drop of Essential Oil of Thyme with a tablespoon of olive oil or coconut oil, or mix it full strength into a pre-made salve. Place on warts daily until the wart is gone.

Harvesting: Harvest thyme leaves often during the summer. Frequent trimming keeps the bushes from becoming woody and increases yield. Use fresh leaves whenever possible and freeze or dry leaves for future use.

Warning: Thyme is safe for use in adults and children. The essential oil is very strong and sometimes causes skin irritations if used full strength. Always dilute the essential oil in a carrier oil before use.

Valerian Root, *Valeriana officinalis*

Valerian is in the Caprifoliaceae (Honeysuckle) Family. There are many species of Valerian, most medicinal, but this is the species most commonly used medicinally. I grow it in my garden and it is my go-to occasional herbal sleep aid. It is also called garden heliotrope and nature's Valium.

Identification: Valerian usually grows from 1 to 5 feet (0.3m to 1.5m) tall depending on the location and the soil conditions. It has a straight round stem that is topped by an umbrella-like flowerhead.

Its opposite dark green leaves have a pinnate blade with 6 to 11 pairs of terminal leaflets. These leaflets have prickly margins and are hairy underneath.

Valerian flowers are in branched batches and each flower is about 1/5 inch long. They are tiny white to pink blossoms. The flower has three stamens and a distinctive scent.

Edible Use: The seeds are edible when lightly roasted.

Medicinal Use: The root is most commonly used but the leaves may also be used for medicine (though they are less potent than the roots).

Insomnia: I use Valerian as a sleep aid with excellent results. People, including myself, report that they get to sleep faster and can sleep longer without waking. They also report that they awaken refreshed without residual drowsiness. It can become habit forming so only use when needed.

Anxiety and Panic Attacks: Valerian root has a calming effect that is beneficial to people with panic and anxiety disorders.

Depression and Obsessive-Compulsive Behavior: Valerian root improves symptoms of depression and obsessive-compulsive disorder (OCD) when used in small doses. In larger doses, it can have the opposite effect.

Epilepsy: Valerian has a relaxing effect on the muscles of the body. For regular use (to prevent attacks), usual dosage is between 100 mg to 1 gram of dried and powdered root.

Start with a low dose, depending on the person's size and the severity of the disease, and increase it gradually until you find a level that works. It can also be used for acute attacks.

Menstrual Cramps: Because of its analgesic properties and its ability to relax the smooth muscles, this herb makes a good treatment for pain and cramping during menstruation.

Lowers Blood Pressure and Pulse Rate: Valerian relaxes the blood vessels to naturally reduce blood pressure and pulse rate.

Quitting Smoking: Valerian root is calming and helps lessen the effects of nicotine withdrawal.

It especially helps with the irritability people often experience when quitting. Use in tincture form.

Harvesting: Cut the flowering tops off as they appear. This enables a better development of the root. In the first year, many of the young plants do not flower but produce a luxuriant crop of leaves. Harvest the roots in autumn. Dig deeply to get the entire root system, planting some back for future harvests. Slice the roots into small sections and dry for future use.

Warning: In ordinary doses, Valerian exerts a quieting and soothing influence upon the brain and nervous system. However, in large repeated doses it can produce pain in the head, heaviness, and stupor. It can become addictive, only use when needed.

Do not use during pregnancy, as its effects are unknown.

Violets, *Viola* spp. including *Viola sororia* (common violet) and *Viola odorata* (sweet violet)

Wild violets are beautiful little plants that are both edible and medicinal. Pansies are also edible. They are in the Violaceae (Violet) Family.

Identification: Wild violets are short plants, usually only 4 to 6 inches (10 cm to 15 cm) high. They grow in clumps with purple, blue, yellow, or white flowers growing on a leafless stalk. Each flower has 5 parts of unequal size. The flowers bloom from early spring into the early summer. Heart-shaped basal leaves grow from its underground root. The leaf margin is toothed but rounded.

These low-growing, perennial plants prefer shady areas, but can grow in sunny locations. The native wildflower favors woods, thickets, and stream banks.

Edible Use: Both the flowers and leaves are edible. Younger leaves and flowers are tender for fresh eating. Older leaves need to be cooked in soups or stews to tenderize them and relieve some of their bitterness. The leaves have a mucilaginous texture that can thicken liquids. Use sweet violets in sweet dishes. The roots and seeds are not eaten and may cause nausea and vomiting.

Freshly picked flowers are beautiful as a garnish in salads, on cakes or pastries, or other foods. Flowers and leaves are rich in vitamins A and C, as well as antioxidants and phytochemicals.

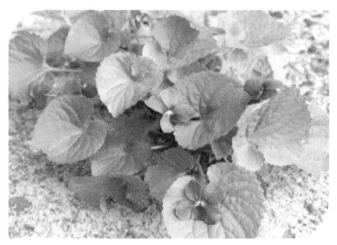

Medicinal Use: Wild violets are an excellent tonic for helping the body detoxify. They strengthen the immune system and stimulate the lymphatic system. They help the body eliminate waste and toxins in the body. Violets are cooling, moistening and relieve pain. They work as a blood cleanser and are safe for elders and children. I use the flowers and leaves internally as a tea or tincture and externally for skin conditions.

Sore Throats, Colds, Sinus Infections, and Other Respiratory Conditions: Wild violets strengthen the immune system and reduce inflammation in the respiratory system. Its mucilaginous properties are useful in soothing the bronchial passages and works as an expectorant to remove mucous from the body. The herb is useful to treat sore throats, colds, sinus infections and other respiratory and bronchial conditions. I like to use Wild Violet Tea for these conditions, but eating the herb is also effective.

Whooping Cough and Dry Hacking Cough: Wild violet has been used for centuries as a bronchial remedy for dry coughs and other bronchial conditions. As a tonic for the lymphatic system and immune system, it helps relieve the underlying problems causing these conditions. Try Wild Violet Tea for coughs.

Anti-inflammatory, Arthritis, and Joint Pain: Wild violets are anti-inflammatory and contain a variety of phytochemicals that are antioxidants and free radical scavengers. Violets can be eaten or taken in tea as an effective anti-inflammatory. The anti-inflammatory effects of wild violet flowers are useful in treating joint pains of all kinds, including the neck and back.

Pound the leaves and flowers to a paste made with a little water, then apply the paste to the skin directly above the painful area. You can cover the poultice with cloth to hold it in place. Use wild violet internally as well as externally for joint pains.

Minor Scrapes and Bruises: Wild violets have antiseptic properties and analgesic properties that relieve the pain while preventing or treating infections and helping the area heal quickly. Use the tea as a wash for areas of skin or apply the flowers as a poultice.

Mild Laxative: Violets have a mild laxative effect and are deemed safe for children.

Lowering Cholesterol and Blood Thinning: The mucilage in violet leaves is helpful in lowering cholesterol levels and in balancing the intestinal flora. The leaves are also high in vitamins A, C, and rutin. Rutin is an antioxidant and anti-inflammatory and has blood thinning properties.

For lowering cholesterol and use as a blood thinner, try eating the leaves, taking leaf powder in capsule form, or using a tea or tincture.

Hemorrhoids and Varicose Veins: The rutin contained in violet leaves is helpful in reducing the inflammation that causes hemorrhoids and varicose veins.

Its mild laxative effect helps prevent straining. You can use a poultice directly on the hemorrhoids or veins or you can apply a salve or infused violet oil.

Skin Conditions, Abrasions, Dermatitis, Insect Bites, Eczema: As an anti-inflammatory and a cooling and soothing herb, wild violet is useful for treating minor skin problems including eczema and other rashes, insect bites and abrasions. Use Wild Violet Tea as a wash on the skin or make a salve or infused oil with the herb for skin use.

Harvesting: I begin harvesting wild violets in April, May, and June when the flowers are freshly opening. The exact time depends on the weather. Once they begin to open, I go back daily to pick what I need.

Gather the petals in the morning while the blooms are fresh. They tend to wilt in the afternoon or in heat. Dry some flowers for use year-round.

Be careful where you gather. Roadsides and parks are often sprayed with pesticides. Look for flowers in pristine areas away from industrial areas, waste areas, and roadsides. Also remember, African Violets are not wild violets and cannot be used.

Warning: Some people get a skin rash on contact with the wild violet leaf. There is no known internal toxicity, but allergies are always possible. Large doses of the roots or seeds can cause severe stomach upset, vomiting, high blood pressure and breathing problems.

Be sure about your identification (if it is in bloom identification is much easier) as there are poisonous look-alikes.

Recipes. Wild Violet Tea: *You can make this tea with all flowers, if you have enough, but 1-part flower to 2 parts leaves works as well. An all-flower recipe makes a milder tasting tea. Ingredients: 2 teaspoons of dried wild violet leaves (or flowers, if desired), 1 teaspoon of dried flowers, 1 cup boiling water, raw honey, optional. Pour the boiling water over the flowers and leaves and allow it to steep for about 5 minutes. Strain the tea and drink. Sweeten with honey, if desired.

NOTE: Do not sweeten the tea if you are using it as a wash on injured skin or for other external use.

White Mustard, *Sinapis alba*

White mustard belongs to the Brassicaceae (Mustard) family. It is mostly grown for its seeds or as fodder crop and is widespread. White mustard seeds are yellow in color and are also called yellow mustard. Brown and black mustards are different but also have medicinal uses.

Identification: White mustard is an annual herb, growing from 1 to 2 feet (0.3m to 0.6m) tall. It flowers from July to September. The white mustard flower has a yellow corolla, just over 1/2 inch (1.25 cm) in diameter with four petals that are 1/4 to 1/2 inch (0.75 cm to 1.25 cm) long. It contains four spreading sepals and six stamens (4 long and two short). The alternate leaves are stalked with a coarsely hairy leaflet. Its stems are branched and also hairy. Each leaf is irregularly pinnately lobed, with irregular sawtooth edges. The terminal leaflets are large and clearly lobed. The fruit of white mustard has many tiny round pale-yellow seeds.

Edible Use: The seeds, flowers, leaves and extracted oil are edible. I like to eat the young leaves in salads, and I sometimes cook the older leaves as a vegetable or potherb. The seeds make a spicy condiment or flavoring when finely ground.

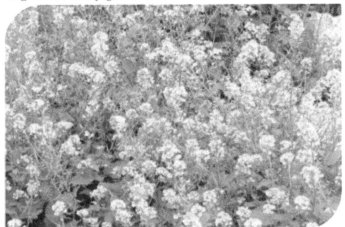

SuperJew, own work, White Mustard near Abu Ghosh.CC 3.0

Medicinal Use: White mustard is antibacterial and antifungal, digestive, diuretic, emetic, expectorant, rubefacient, and stimulant. It is used internally and externally.

Pneumonia, Bronchitis, Respiratory Diseases: The seeds of white mustard, powdered and made into a poultice, are good for treating respiratory diseases. They act as an irritant to loosen phlegm and help expel mucus from the body. The poultice is applied to the chest and left in place until the skin reddens, then promptly removed. The mustard is an irritant and can cause blistering if left in place too long.

Poison Ingestion: Ground mustard seed, taken by mouth in quantity, can cause vomiting. You can use it to bring up poisons and other undesirable substances that have been ingested.

Preventing Infection: To prevent infection in a wound, or anywhere in the body, white mustard is a good ally. It has abundant sulfur compounds, which help prevent infection and fight any invading infection. Often used in combination with garlic. For best effects, use fresh mustard seeds, ground into a paste. When using dried mustard seeds, soak them in water before grinding them.

Prevents Cancer: Mustard seeds contain beneficial substances that reduce the risk and the reoccurrence of cancer. It does not cure cancer, but seems to prevent the spread or the return of it. One tablespoon of crushed or ground white mustard seed daily is enough to provide these powerful benefits.

Arthritis: White mustard applied to the skin is an irritant. The skin irritation brings an increased blood supply to the area. The skin and joints are warmed, and pain is reduced. You must be careful to wash the mustard away once the skin reddens to prevent blisters and other damage to the skin.

To treat arthritis and other joint pain, mix ground white mustard seeds with enough vinegar to make a paste. Apply to the skin over the affected area. White mustard seed powder (1 tablespoon) added to the bath water is also beneficial for arthritic pain.

Sore Throats: Mustard Seed Tea made from the leaves of the white mustard plant has a beneficial effect on sore throats. The increased blood circulation and sulfur content help the throat to heal. Gargle Mustard Seed Tea several times daily, beginning at the first sign of throat irritation. Its action is similar to that of a cayenne gargle.

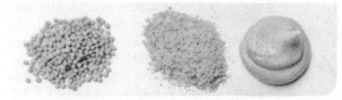

Chilblains (Chill Burns): Chilblains benefit from the warming power of white mustard. Mix one-part white mustard seed powder and four parts ground flax seeds together to make a paste. Use this mixture as a poultice to get rid of chilblains.

Recipes: Mustard Seed Tea. You need 1 teaspoon crushed mustard seeds and 1 cup boiling water. Pour the water over the mustard seeds and let it steep covered for 2 to 4 minutes.

Yellow Mustard Poultice. You'll need: one tablespoon ground white mustard seeds, 1/2 cup flour, 1 egg white, 8 ounces (250ml) of hot water. Mix the mustard and flour together, then add the egg white and water to form a loose paste. Apply immediately to the body over the affected area.

Wild Lettuce, *Lactuca canadensis, L. virosa* and *L. serriola*

This member of the Daisy/Aster Family is very widespread. Its sap is well known for pain relief. Most *Lactuca* species of wild lettuce contain these pain-relieving lactones in their milky latex. It is also known as prickly lettuce and opium lettuce (although it does not actually contain opium).

Identification: Wild lettuce grows to be 3 to 5 feet (0.9m to 1.5m) tall, usually on a single stem, and has a milky sap throughout the root, leaves, and stems. The central stem is light-green to reddish-green, occasionally with purple streaks. Its green alternating leaves sometimes have purple edges or a yellowish color.

The lance-shaped leaves can grow up to 3 inches (7.5 cm) across and 10 inches (25 cm) long. Leaves are usually, but not always, lobed and look similar to a dandelion leaf. Some species have spines/prickly hairs along the midrib on the underside of the leaf and some have teeth on their leaf margins that are very prickly.

The white milky sap turns tan after exposure to air. This is an important diagnostic feature. Wild lettuce blooms in the late summer to early autumn. Its flowers are small and are similar to dandelions with yellow or slightly reddish - orange petals. Flower heads are much smaller than those of dandelion - about 1/3 inch (0.8

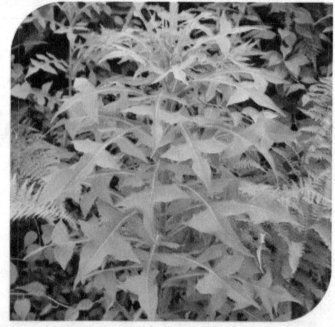

Photo:http://extension.umass.edu/landscape/weeds/lactuca-canadensis

cm) across with 12 to 25 rays – and they are well above the leaves on a tall stem, unlike dandelion, whose flowers are low to the ground. After 3 to 4 weeks, the flowers are replaced with dark brown, dry fruits with white hairs. The taproot is thick and deep.

Edible Use: This slightly bitter lettuce is good to eat when the leaves are cooked like spinach. Boiling removes some of its bitterness. It can be eaten raw, but is usually too bitter for most people's tastes.

Medicinal Use: The white latex sap that runs through the plant contains sesquiterpene lactones,

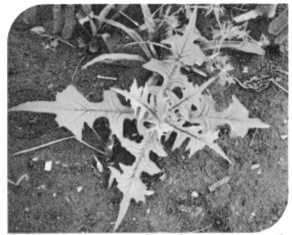

which are its primary medicinal components, similar to Chicory (also in this book). Older plants have higher concentrations of sap, especially while the plant is just beginning to bloom. Best to use the sap after it dries or use a tincture form to make full use of its medicinal compounds.

Insomnia and Sedative: The sedative properties of wild lettuce come from the milky sap that runs through the stems and leaves. It calms restlessness and anxiety and induces sleep without being addictive.

Pain Relief and Shock: Wild lettuce has also been called opium lettuce because of its weak opium-like effects. Used in small doses, it has a sedative and pain-relieving effect without causing the stomach upset and high of a true opium. It is also helpful in the treatment of shock, menstrual pain, muscular pain, joints pain, and colic.

Warts: Apply the white sap to the skin as a treatment for external warts. Cover the wart with sap once or twice a day until the wart is gone.

Warning: Use with caution as it has a sedative effect. Do not overdose.

Harvesting: Collect the leaves and stems in the summer when the plant is just starting to bloom for maximum medicinal properties. Even better is to simply collect the milky sap directly into a small glass jar. This is more time-consuming but gives you the most concentrated dose. The sap turns brown and hardens when dry. Older plants are best. Leave behind enough of the plant so that it will recover.

Recipes. Wild Lettuce Tincture: You will need: vodka, brandy or other 80 proof alcohol, fresh or dried wild lettuce leaves. Fill a clean, sterile, glass jar with chopped fresh milky leaves or use 2 ounces (56g) of dried wild lettuce per cup of alcohol. You may also use the sap. Cover the herbs with vodka or other drinkable alcohol. Stir the herbs to remove air bubbles. Move the container to a cool, dark place and allow the tincture to steep for 3 to 4 weeks, shaking daily. Strain out the herbs and discard. Store in a cool, dark place for up to 5 years.

Wild Teasel, *Dipsacus sylvestris/ fullonum*

Also known as Fuller's Teasel, Wild Teasel, or Common Teasel, this plant grows throughout most of the United States and coastal Canada. It is listed as a noxious weed in many states, but it has many good uses. Teasel grows in large patches, crowding out other plants once established. In the fall, it attracts large flocks of birds, who use the seeds as a winter food source. It likes to grow along stream banks, roadsides, pastureland, prairies, meadows, savannas, and woodland borders. It is a water loving plant that grows in a variety of soils including sandy soils in moist areas and heavy clay in poorly drained areas. It is in the Caprifoliaceae, the honeysuckle family.

Identification: Teasel is a biennial herbaceous plant. It has lance shaped leaves and grows from 3 to 8 feet in height. The first-year leaves form a rosette at the base of the stem with the flower stem emerging from the center in the second year. Each leaf is 8 to 16 inches (20 cm-40 cm) long and 1 to 2.5 inches (2.5 cm to 6 cm) across. The underside of the leaf has a row of spines along the midrib and the stems are also covered in small spines. The plant has a two-year

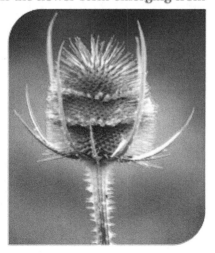

lifecycle, growing leaves and stems in the first year and producing flowers in the second year. It has erect hollow pale green to reddish-green stems. Its stems are hairless with longitudinal ridges and white spines.

Teasel flowers June through August. It has a cylindrical inflorescence of dark pink, purple, or lavender flowers on the top of the flower stem. The inflorescence is ovoid or conical, up to 4 inches long (10cm) and 2 inches (5cm) across. When the flowers drop, the flower cylinder dries into spiny hard bracts with small seeds maturing mid-autumn.

The plant has a deep taproot with fibrous secondary roots that can grow up to 2 feet long (0.6m) and up to an inch (2.5cm) in diameter.

Edible Use: The young leaves are edible, but the short hairs make them unappetizing. They can be eaten cooked or raw. The roots are used medicinally but are not eaten.

Non-Edible Use: A water-soluble blue dye, used as an indigo substitute, is obtained from the plant. When the plant is mixed with alum, a yellow dye is obtained.

The stalks work as a spindle for friction fire, and can be paired with a clematis fireboard.

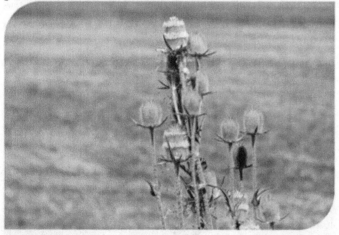

Medicinal Use: Teasel root can be taken internally and externally, but you must be very careful with internal dosing, especially if you have, or suspect you have, Lyme Disease. For Lyme, I prefer to use teasel in a tincture form with a maximum dose of 9 drops split into 3 drops each in the morning, afternoon, and evening. Begin by taking 1 drop in the morning of the first day. On the second day, take one drop in the morning and one in the evening. On the third day, take one drop in the morning, afternoon, and evening. Continue adding one drop each day until you reach the maximum of 9

drops total each day (three in the morning, three in the afternoon, and three in the evening.) Note that you may have a Jarisch-Herxheimer ("herx")" reaction if you have Lyme. A "herx" reaction is an adverse response to the cytokines that are released as the Lyme bacteria are killed. Once the bacterial waste and dead bacteria are expelled this reaction goes away. This does mean that the spirochaetes that cause Lyme are dying, which is good news, but you may feel worse before you feel better.

Personally, I use teasel tincture in larger amounts as a Lyme preventative when I am in an area with Lyme-carrying deer ticks (see "Lyme Prevention" below).

Treats Chronic Lyme Disease: Lyme disease is a bacterial infection of the spirochete Borrelia burgdorferi and is transmitted by infected deer/black-legged (Ixodes spp.) ticks. The spirochaetes drill into human tissue and, in time, seal themselves in by creating a biofilm, which acts as a barrier to antibiotics.

Teasel is not an antibiotic, but it acts to boost the effectiveness of antibiotics, dumping the bacteria back into the blood stream where antibiotics can more easily attack and clear the infection. In most cases, antibiotics given soon after infection work well for Lyme, but in the case of Chronic Lyme Disease, where antibiotics are not working well enough, adding teasel to the cure can make all the difference. It may still take 6 months or longer to clear the infection, but the teasel is thought to draw the spirochaetes out of the tissue, thus exposing them to the antibiotics. Please see suggested dosing instructions above.

Lyme Prevention: I use teasel tincture as a Lyme preventative when I am in an area with Lyme-carrying ticks. I take a dropperful 2x/day if I am in the woods in a known Lyme area. I know many other people who work in the woods who also use teasel in this way. It keeps Borrelia from burrowing into my tissues in case of an infection. If you do get a tick bite save the tick to get it tested for Lyme. If antibiotics are taken early Lyme can be prevented.

Osteoporosis, Osteopenia, and Bone Fractures: Teasel root increases blood circulation so that the body can rebuild and repair tendons and bones. It stimulates new bone growth and helps increase bone mass. It is an effective treatment for both Osteoporosis and Osteopenia and for bone fractures once the bone has been properly set.

Natural Diuretic: Teasel root is excellent at ridding the body of excess water and encouraging urine flow. Teasel rids the body of unnecessary water weight, salt, and toxins.

It helps reduce inflammation and swelling and can be useful in reducing a fever by stimulating sweating.

Candida and Yeast Infections: Teasel root works to purge excess yeast and Candida from the body into the bloodstream where it dies and is eliminated. Teasel is useful in keeping yeast infections and Candida under control.

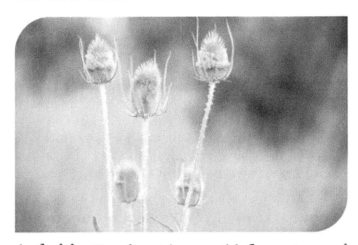

Arthritis: Teasel root is an anti-inflammatory and helps repair damaged joints that cause arthritis. It gives some short-term pain relief, but it takes long-term use for effective arthritis relief.

Jaundice and Liver Problems: Teasel is a liver tonic, and is helpful in treating liver problems of many types, including jaundice.

The diuretic properties of teasel root support the liver and help clear the body of the toxins that cause jaundice. It supports the liver and helps reduce inflammation and infections, but it does not cure the underlying cause.

Wounds and Inflammation – External Application: For skin wounds and inflammation, teasel root powder can be sprinkled directly on the affected site. To use, grind dried teasel root into a fine powder and apply or add water to make a poultice.

Harvesting Teasel: I recommend wearing gloves and protective clothing to protect your skin from the teasel spines. Harvest the roots after the end of the first year's growth between early autumn and early spring. Once they have flower stalks it is too late, as the roots become woody.

Dig up the plant with a spading fork, pushing deeply into the soil next to the plant. The taproot is deep with additional secondary roots. Wiggle the fork to loosen the soil and push it as deep as possible. Grab the plant with a gloved hand and pull the plant up, loosening more with the spading fork as needed.

Take enough teasel root to make a year's supply of tincture at once. Wash them, slice them and cut away the brown parts, tough roots, or soft roots. You want to use the center of the root. Use fresh root to make tincture or place them in the dehydrator to dry for powder or future use. Make sure to cut them before they dry out, as they are very difficult to cut once they are dry.

Warning: Take care in dosing teasel root tincture, starting with one drop only and slowly increasing it as tolerated.

Teasel root can cause a "herx" reaction in some people (see "Lyme" section above). These side effects subside over time.

Fresh Teasel Root Tincture Recipe: Fresh teasel root, sliced and chopped into small pieces, 100 proof vodka or similar proof drinking alcohol, 2 clean jars with tight-fitting lids, Strainer. Use the center of the fresh root for this recipe. Place the chopped root in a clean jar, filling it to within one inch of the top. Cover it with 100 proof alcohol, completely filling the jar to the rim.

Cap it tightly and label /date the jar. Shake the jar weekly. Refill with 100 proof alcohol if needed. Allow the tincture to macerate for 6 to 8 weeks, then strain and move it to a clean jar. Store Teasel Tincture in a cool, dark place for up to 5 years.

Dose Teasel Tincture carefully, starting with 1 drop and increasing by 1 drop daily to a maximum of 9 drops total daily if using for Lyme. Divide the doses into morning, afternoon, and night doses, never giving more than 3 drops per dose.

Wooly Lamb's Ear, *Stachys byzantina*

Wooly Lamb's Ear was used in WWII as a field dressing for wounds on the battlefield. It is easy to cultivate in the garden in full sun. It is also known as wooly wound wort, wooly betony and silver carpet. It is in the Lamiaceae (Mint) Family.

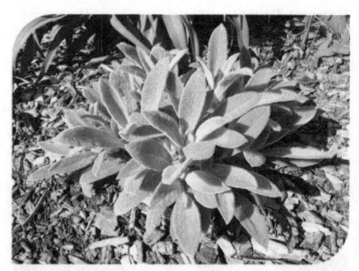

Identification: This perennial plant has soft, fuzzy leaves that are densely covered with silver-white or gray hairs with the texture of velvet. Leaves have a curved shape and are 2 to 4 inches (5 cm to 10 cm) long with a rounded point. The undersides are more silvery-white in color than the tops. Flowering stems grow erect, with square stems, and are usually 1 to 2 feet (0.3 meters to 0.6 meters) tall. The flowering spikes are 4 to 10 inches (10 cm to 15 cm) long with many purple flowers crowded together on the stem. Small leaves appear on the flowering stems as well. The crushed plant has a pleasant scent, mildly like apple or pineapple.

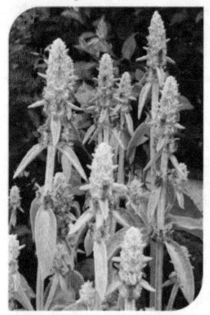

Wolly Lamb's Ear, Jean-Pol ANDMONT, CC by SA 3.0

Edible and Other Use: The leaves are edible and best when young and tender. Eat them fresh in salads or steam them as a green vegetable. Wooly Lamb's Ear is soft and very absorbent, which makes it a good substitute for toilet paper. The highly absorbent properties of the leaves make it useful as a feminine hygiene product too.

Medicinal Use: Lamb's Ear is antibacterial, antiseptic, antispasmodic, and astringent. It is also a diuretic, febrifuge, good for digestion, styptic, tonic, vermifuge, and wound-healing.

Wound Dressing: The soft, fuzzy leaves of Lamb's Ear make an excellent dressing for wounds of all kinds. They are antibacterial, antiseptic, and anti-inflammatory and are said to combat MRSA. The leaves absorb blood and encourage clotting. Place several whole leaves on the wound and cover it with a soft cloth or gauze. Leave in place until it is time to change the dressing.

Wound Wash, Eye Wash, Conjunctivitis, and Sties: Make a medicinal tea to use as an eyewash. When cool, the tea makes an excellent antibacterial wash for wounds of all kinds. When using it as an eyewash or to treat pinkeye, make the tea with distilled water and bring it to a full boil. Then strain it twice to make sure no fine particles remain.

Diarrhea, Fevers, and Internal Bleeding: Wooly Lamb's Ear works for internal bleeding, for diarrhea, and for reducing fevers. For these purposes, drink Wooly Lamb's Ear Tea (recipe found below).

Sore Mouth and Sore Throat: The same tea, used as a gargle, is effective for treating a sore throat or mouth. Swish the tea around in the mouth or gargle with it several times a day. It relieves the pain and the antibiotic properties help cure the underlying infection.

Liver and Heart Tonic: The healthful benefits of Wooly Lamb's Ear make it a good general tonic, especially for the liver and heart. Take the tea daily or consume the leaves as an herb or vegetable.

Insect Bites and Hemorrhoids: The anti-inflammatory benefits of lamb's ear make it effective in dealing with painful bee stings and insect bites. It also has some analgesic properties, which help with pain.

Recipes. Wooly Lamb's Ear Tea: You will only need fresh leaves of Wooly Lamb's Ear and water. Bruise the fresh leaves by pounding then add them to

a pot of simmering water. Simmer the leaves for a 5 to 10 minutes and cool. Strain the liquid through a fine sieve or coffee filter to remove all leaf particles. Drink or use as a wash.

Yarrow,
Achillea millefolium

I always keep yarrow in my medicine bag, as it has many uses. It is also called nosebleed plant, squirrel's tale, plumajillo, and soldier's woundwort. I recognize it by its feathery leaf shape, texture, and scent. It is in the Aster/Daisy Family. It is found in temperate zones throughout the world.

Identification: Yarrow is an erect plant that grows from a spreading rhizome. The plant has finely divided feathery leaves that grow along the stem. Plants grow 1 to 3 feet (0.3m to 0.9 meters) in full sun to partial shade. Its bipinnate or tripinnate leaves are 2 to 8 inches (5 cm to 20 cm) long, and can be hairy. Leaves are arranged spirally on the stem in groups of 2 to 3. Each leaf is divided into many leaflets, which are further divided into smaller leaflets. The silvery-green leaves are fern-like and feathery.

Flowers bloom from May to July. Each inflorescence is a cluster of 15 to 40 tiny disk flowers surrounded by 3 to 8 ray flowers. The scent of yarrow is similar to chrysanthemums, and the flowers are very long lasting. Colors range from white to yellow, pink, and red. Yarrow is a good companion plant in a garden, as it repels many garden pests while attracting beneficial insects.

Edible Use: You can eat the leaves raw or cooked. They are bitter and are best eaten young. The plant is very nutritious; however, I don't recommend eating a lot of it because of its blood clotting ability.

The flowers and leaves are used to make tea, but the leaf tea is bitter. A little raw honey helps.

Medicinal Use: All parts of the plant are used medicinally.

Stopping Internal & External Bleeding: Yarrow quickly stops bleeding by contracting the blood vessels and encouraging clotting. Yarrow contains anti-inflammatory and antibacterial compounds that ease swelling and promote healing. It also helps disinfect wounds. If it is possible, clean the wound before applying yarrow. Yarrow will quickly stop bleeding and bind any dirt or infectious materials into the wound, so best to clean first if possible.

To use yarrow leaves on a wound or abscess, chop or rip the leaves finely and apply to the wound. I often carry dried powdered yarrow with me for this purpose. Cover the wound with a soft cloth and leave it in place. Repeat 2 to 3 times daily until the wound is healed over and the swelling is gone. Yarrow oil or tincture can be used to treat nosebleeds and other minor injuries, as can yarrow powder. Place a few drops of oil or tincture on the affected area or apply it to a tissue or cloth and place it on the wound.

Bruises, Sprains, Swelling, and Hemorrhoids: For bruises, sprains, hemorrhoids, and other swellings, use a poultice of yarrow leaves or stems pounded into a paste and applied to the injured area and cover. Infused yarrow oil or salve works well for bruises, sprains, swelling, and hemorrhoids.

Antibacterial and Antifungal: Yarrow is a strong antibacterial and antifungal. It will heal a wound quickly. Do not use on deep puncture wounds as it will heal it too quickly and you want the wound to heal from the inside out. It is a great addition to a first aid salve. It is also a strong antifungal.

Fevers, Colds, and Measles: Yarrow reduces the duration of the measles virus, colds, and fevers. It is quick to bring down a fever. Either chew raw yarrow or drink yarrow tea to induce sweating and reduce fevers.

An easier (and more palatable) method is to take yarrow in tincture form. It opens the pores, encouraging perspiration, and purifies and moves the blood.

Menstrual Problems: Yarrow tea or tincture treats menstrual problems ranging from a lack of menstruation to excessive bleeding and cramping. It tones the uterine muscles after childbirth, reduces cramping by relaxing the smooth muscles, and prevents hemorrhage. It also helps to bring on menses.

Dental Pain: To reduce inflammation and relieve dental pain, chew on a piece of fresh yarrow root or yarrow leaves. In addition to its anti-inflammatory and anti-infection benefits, yarrow contains salicylic acid, a pain reliever that acts quickly.

Mastitis: As an antibacterial and an anti-inflammatory yarrow works well for mastitis. A leaf poultice seems to work the best while alternating between warm and cold compresses (cabbage leaves also work well for mastitis).

Anxiety and Relaxation without Sedation: Yarrow seems to reduce anxiety without sedative effects. It has a calming effect on the central nervous system.

Harvesting: Yarrow is best when young, picked in the spring or early summer before the flowers have been pollinated. Dry the leaves, stems, and flowers for later use. Once the herb is dry, store it in a capped jar in a cool, dark, and dry location.

Warning: Do not eat yarrow or take yarrow tea during pregnancy. Some people are allergic to yarrow. Do not use it if you are allergic to plants in the Aster/Daisy family, if you develop a rash, or if any irritation occurs. Do not use before surgery.

Recipes. Yarrow Tea: One teaspoon dried yarrow flowers and/or leaves, one cup boiling water, sweetener, if desired. Pour one cup of boiling water over one teaspoon of dried yarrow flowers or leaves. Cover and allow the tea to steep for 5 minutes. Sweeten with raw honey or maple syrup.

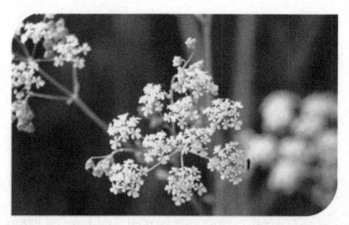

Yarrow Tincture: Ingredients: fresh yarrow leaves and flowers, vodka, brandy, or other alcohol, 80 proof or higher. Chop yarrow into small pieces and pack it tightly to fill a glass jar. Fill the jar with alcohol and cover it tightly. Check the jar every few days and add more alcohol as needed to keep the jar full. Allow the tincture to steep for 6 to 8 weeks. Strain the alcohol through a few layers of cheesecloth and squeeze out all the liquid. Discard the herbs, label the jar and store your tincture in a cool, dark place.

Yarrow Oil: Fresh or dried yarrow leaves, organic olive oil or another carrier oil. If using fresh yarrow, cut the leaves into one-inch (2.5 cm) pieces and allow them to dry. Place the herbs into a jar or heatproof container and add oil just to cover the herbs. Fill a small pot about 1/3 full of water and bring to a boil. Turn the heat down to a simmer before using. Place the jar of oil and herbs into the water, preventing the water from getting into the oil container. Use the water like a double-boiler to gently heat the herbs and oil for 2 to 3 hours. Do not overheat! Allow the oil to cool, then filter it through a couple of layers of cheesecloth. Squeeze the cheesecloth to get all the oil. Discard the herb and use the oil for medicinal purposes.

Yarrow Salve: Ingredients: ½ cup (4 oz or 125ml)) Infused Yarrow Oil, 1-ounce Beeswax. Using a double boiler, mix the beeswax and the infused oil until the beeswax has melted. Check the consistency by dipping a spoon in and putting it in the fridge to harden. If it is not hard enough, add more beeswax. If too hard add more oil. Pour into your jar or tins and let harden. Label and date.

Forest, Scrublands, and Woodlands

Amaranthus caudatus

Amaranthus caudatus is a brilliantly beautiful plant. Its tails of bright red flowers make it easy to locate, even at a distance. It is also called loves-lies-bleeding, tassel flower, velvet flower, foxtail amaranth, pendant amaranth, and quilete. It is in the Amaranthaceae (Amaranth) Family. *Amaranthus caudatus* is widespread throughout North America. It often grows in disturbed ground.

Identification: *Amaranthus caudatus* is an annual flowering plant. It grows from 3 to 8 feet (0.9m to 2.4m) tall in full sun with a spread of 1 to 3 feet (0.3m to 0.9m). It blooms from July until the first frost. The red flowers are very small and have no petals. They bloom in drooping terminal tassel-like panicles that are 1 to 2 feet (0.3m to 0.6m) long. The seeds ripen in September.

Edible Use: The leaves and seeds of *Amaranthus caudatus* are edible. Amaranth leaves can be eaten raw or cooked. The seeds are used as a grain. They do not need to be cooked, but are good toasted in a little oil. The seeds are also good when sprouted.

Medicinal Use: The plant is astringent, anti-parasitic, and diuretic.

Diabetes: People with diabetes can substitute Amaranthus for rice and also eat the seeds and leaves as often as possible. It has anti-diabetic properties that help regulate blood sugar and brings it down significantly.

Lowers Cholesterol: Amaranthus seeds and oil are a healthy choice for those with hypertension, cardiovascular disease, and high cholesterol.

Sore Throats, Mouth Sores, and Canker Sores: A gargle made from dried and powdered Amaranthus leaves is an effective treatment for sore throats and canker sores. To make a gargle, boil 2 tablespoons of powdered amaranth leaves in 1 cup of

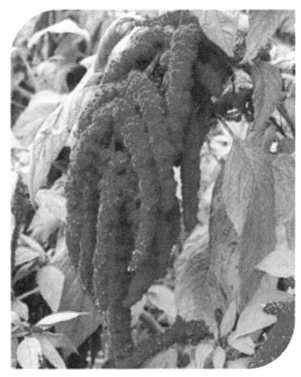

Amaranthus caudatus, Tubifex, CC by SA 3.0

water for 10 minutes. Let it cool and gargle and swish with it three or more times a day.

Heavy Menstrual Bleeding and Stopping Bleeding: *Amaranthus caudatus* is a powerful blood clotting agent and works to stop excess menstrual bleeding. Boil 1 tablespoon of root powder in 1 cup of water. Let it cool, then consume. For external bleeding, dust the affected area with the root powder. It quickly stops nosebleeds and bleeding from other small wounds.

Vaginal Infections: Use an Amaranthus leaf and root powder decoction internally, and use externally as a douche to treat vaginal discharge.

Warning: *Amaranthus caudatus* should not be used by people who have gout, rheumatoid arthritis, or kidney disorders. It should not be given to pregnant women, nursing mothers, or babies.

American Ginseng, *Panax quinquefolius*

American ginseng, also known as *Panax ginseng*, is in the Araliaceae (Ginseng/Ivy) Family. It is native to eastern North America and cultivated widely elsewhere. Its aromatic root forks as it matures.

Identification: Plants grow 6 to 18 inches (15 cm to 45 cm) tall. Its leaves are palmate and divided into 3 to 7 (usually 4 or 5) lance-shaped, sharp-toothed leaflets. The flowers are whitish-greenish, and fruits are pea-sized red berries with two seeds each.

The neck of the rhizome shows scars left by each year's growth. Counting the leaf scars ages the root. Its medicinal compounds, called ginsenosides, increase in concentration as the root ages. In general, harvest roots 4 years or older.

Medicinal Use: *Panax* species have a well-deserved reputation as powerful adaptogens. They help the body recover from the effects of stress and adrenal fatigue, much like Reishi or Ashwagandha. It is also used as an aphrodisiac and for erectile disfunction. American ginseng is a relaxant, while the Asian version, *P. ginseng*, is said to be more stimulating. The mature root and leaves can be chewed, powdered and put into capsules, extracted in alcohol as a tincture, or made into a tea.

Diabetes: Ginseng has many benefits for diabetics. American ginseng helps regulate blood sugar. Taking take 2 to 5 drops of American Ginseng tincture before each meal helps prevent post-meal spikes in blood sugar levels. It is recommended starting with 2 drops

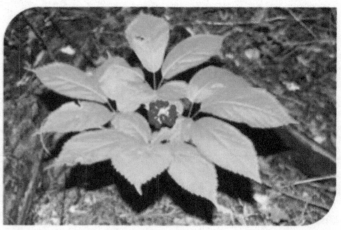
Photo by John Carl Jacobs, CC by SA 4.0

and monitoring blood sugar levels. Increase the dosage one drop at a time, as needed, up to 5 drops per meal, depending on the potency of your tincture. American ginseng contains a class of compounds called ginsenosides, which possess antioxidant and anti-inflammatory properties, two important factors in the progression of diabetes. American ginseng also promotes the secretion of insulin, necessary for regulation of blood sugar levels.

Ginseng helps lower high blood pressure in diabetics. Regular use gives some protection to the heart and retina from diabetes-induced damage.

Cold and Flu: American Ginseng helps fight the common cold and flu when taken regularly. People who take ginseng daily report fewer colds and less severe cold and flu symptoms.

Tonic for Fatigue, Stress, Memory, and Concentration: American ginseng has properties that boost energy and stamina and reduces fatigue caused by failing health and everyday stresses. It also betters cognitive performance, and enhances memory.

Erectile Dysfunction: American ginseng is an effective treatment for erectile dysfunction when taken on a regular basis. Favorable results are only seen when the herb is taken daily over the long term. It seems to work by opening up necessary blood vessels for improved blood flow.

Other Uses for American Ginseng: Since *Panax* is a tonic and reduces the stress on the body, it is effective for use in many different diseases and conditions. It is said to raise the spirits and to improve sleep, mood, and general outlook on life. It is also an antispasmodic.

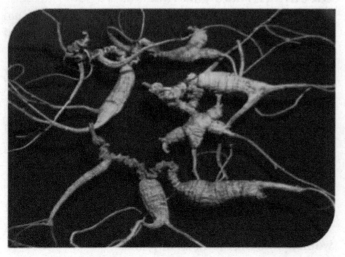

Harvesting: Like all plants, the ginseng root needs to be treated with great respect. Do not harvest the roots before the berries ripen and the seeds set, in late summer or early autumn. When uncovering the neck of the root, look for four or more leaf scars, one scar for each year of age. Roots less than four years old do not contain enough beneficial properties to be effective. Note the location of younger roots and leave them in the ground or dig them up for relocation. The root branches underground, so dig carefully, and excavate a large area. Use the root fresh and dry some for future use.

Warning: Avoid American Ginseng if taking warfarin or other blood thinning therapies. Not recommended for pregnant or breastfeeding women. Ginseng should not be taken if someone has a hormone-related condition such as endometriosis, fibroids, or cancers of the breast, ovaries, uterus, or prostate. Do not use ginseng for people with heart disease except under the close supervision of a healthcare professional. Ginseng may decrease the rate and force of heartbeats.

Occasional side effects include headaches, anxiety, upset stomach, and sometimes trouble sleeping.

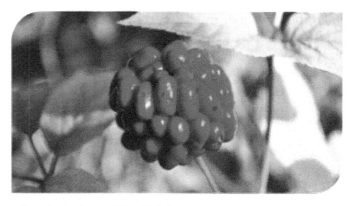

Photo by Drginseng, CC by SA 3.0

Recipes. American Ginseng Tea: Here is a simple ginseng tea with cooling properties. It keeps the body balanced and improves mental alertness. Avoid taking ginseng tea close to bedtime. You'll need 1/2 ounce of American Ginseng root fibers, 3 cups of water, a few grains of salt (optional). Bring the water to a boil. Add ginseng and simmer for 5 to 10 minutes. Season with salt, if desired. Strain the tea and allow it to cool. Serve at room temperature or cold.

American Ginseng Extract: See Section on Tinctures and Extracts. Use 8 ounces (230g) of American ginseng root, pounded into fibers or ground, with 1-quart (1 Liter) of 80 proof or better alcohol and infuse it for 6 to 8 weeks.

Angelica,
Angelica archangelica

According to legend, an angel revealed in a dream how to use angelica to cure the plague. It was reverently called "The Root of the Holy Ghost" and was believed to ward off witchcraft and evil spirits. It is also called Wild Celery.

Angelica is a useful medicinal plant, but care must be taken to identify the plant correctly before using it. It is similar in appearance to other poisonous plants like water hemlock and giant hogweed. Please note the distinguishing features listed below and be sure you have the correct plant before harvesting.

The plant is found in the North Eastern parts of North America and in Northern Europe and grows in moist, cool woodlands, along stream banks, and in shady places. It is widely cultivated as an ornamental and medicinal plant. There are many varieties, but it is the

Angelica archangelica that is used medicinally. It is in the Apiaceae/Umbelliferae (Carrot/Celery) Family.

Identification: Angelica is a biennial plant that dies after it sets its seed in its second year. During the first

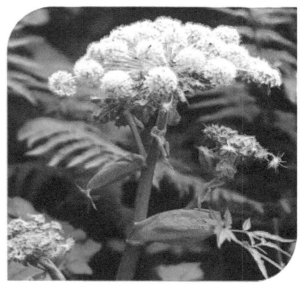

Photo By H. Zell, CC by SA 3.0

year, the plant puts out leaves, but most of its growth and its flowering stage occurs in the second year. It grows from 4 to 6 feet (1.2m – 1.8m) tall and occasionally up to 10 feet tall (3m), with large dark green bipinnate leaves. Each leaf contains many leaflets, divided into three main groups.

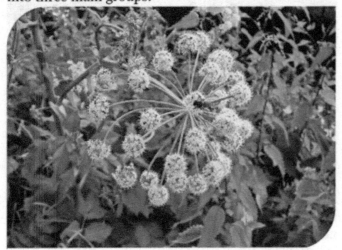

Photo By Franz Xaver, CC by SA 3.0

Each subdivision is further divided into three groups. The leaves are finely serrated. The lower leaves are the largest, up to 2 feet wide (0.6m). The leaf stalks are flattened and fluted. Stems are curved inward with sheathing that forms an elongated bowl that holds water. Stems are dark purple, round, smooth and hollow and are 1 to 2 inches (2.5cm-5cm) across.

The small, plentiful white, yellowish, or greenish-white flowers grow in large, compound umbels, up to 6 inches wide (15cm). The star-shaped flowers appear in July after the second year.

The fruit are small, oblong and pale yellow. Each is 1/6 to 1/4 inch (0.4cm – 0.6cm) in length when ripe and they reside in round heads that are up to 8 to 10 inches (20cm – 25cm) in diameter.

The root is branched, thick, and fleshy with small rootlets. The root is 3 to 6 inches (7.5cm – 15 cm) long.

Edible Use: The fresh root is rumored to be poisonous, but cooked and crystalized pieces of root and stem are used as decorative pieces for cakes and are used for flavoring in alcoholic beverages.

Young shoots and leaves are edible raw or cooked. The flavor is sweet and similar to celery with a slight licorice taste. Use the shoots in salads or boil them like a pot herb. Use angelica stems when young and tender.

Preserve them in sugar or candy them for use as a decoration on sweet treats.

Angelica root must be dried and preserved for later use. Do not use it fresh.

Medicinal Use: The entire plant is used medicinally. Leaves, stems, and flowers are crushed and used in a bath or as a poultice. The medicine from the roots is best extracted using alcoholic tinctures. Roots can be dried and powdered for medicinal use.

Respiratory Issues: The herb is well known as an expectorant and is used to treat bronchitis, asthma, colic, coughs, and the common cold. The root is best used for respiratory ailments, but stems and seeds are also usable when necessary. A tincture or a tea will work as an expectorant.

Digestive Aid, Stimulates Appetite, and Intestinal Infections: Angelica stimulates the appetite, improves digestion, soothes colic, and reduces the production of intestinal gas. It also increases the production of stomach acid. It has been used as a cure for the plague, dysentery, cholera and intestinal infections. The herb is anti-bacterial and kills the bacteria that cause many gastric illnesses, like E. coli.

Nerve Pain: Rub angelica directly on the skin to treat neuralgia or nerve pain. It acts as an anesthetic.

Joint Pain: The anti-inflammatory properties of Angelica are useful for treating arthritis, gout, swelling, and for broken bones. For joint pain, a poultice made from crushed leaves is effective.

Anti-Seizure Effects: Recent studies show that Angelica archangelica protects the body against chemically induced seizures. Angelica essential oil exhibits

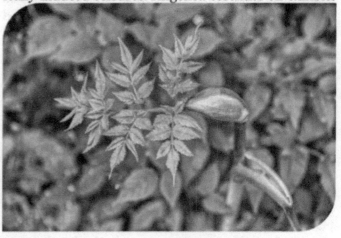

anti-seizure effects, probably due to the presence of terpenes in the oil.

Sore Throats and Mouth Sores: The antibacterial and anti-inflammatory properties of the root is useful in treating sore throats and mouth sores. Use an Angelica Infusion as a gargle or wash several times a day.

Menstrual Problems: Angelica regulates female hormones, regulates the menstrual cycle, and controls menstrual discharge.

Acne: Anti-bacterial and anti-inflammatory compounds in angelica help prevent and control acne. Use an angelica decoction or angelica tea as a face wash.

Anxiety: Recent studies showed that angelica has an antidepressant and anti-anxiety effect. It reduces stress and improves relaxation.

Cancer: Angelica archangelica has been shown to be effective against breast cancer cells. It reduces proliferation of the cancer cells and reduces tumor growth. Research is ongoing into its anti-tumor properties.

Anti-Fungal: Powdered angelica root is used to treat athlete's foot and other fungal infections.

Improves Circulation: Angelica strengthens the heart and improves blood circulation throughout the body.

Harvesting: While all the parts of the herb are useable for culinary and medicinal purposes, they are useable only during certain parts of the year. The roots are best harvested in the fall or winter of the first year. The stem and leaves are best in the spring or early summer of the second year, before the flowers appear. Dry the roots at or below 95 F and store in an airtight container.

Warning: Some people are allergic to Angelica. Avoid using angelica with anti-coagulant drugs. Do not use during pregnancy or breastfeeding. People with Diabetes should not use Angelica

Recipes. Angelica Tea or Decoction: Add 1/2 teaspoon of powdered angelica root to one cup of boiling water. Simmer for 10 to 15 minutes. Turn off the heat and let the tea steep for another 8 to 10 minutes. Strain out the root and store the decoction in a glass jar for later use. Use as a wash for skin problems or drink a cup after meals.

Candied Angelica: Trim angelica shoots and cut into strips. Blanch the strips in boiling water, then cook them in sugar syrup, gradually increasing the amount of sugar. Dry them and store in a sealed container. Keep the syrup for other uses.

Arnica cordifolia, Heartleaf Arnica and *A. montana*

Heartleaf arnica, also known as mountain tobacco, is one of the many Arnica species used for medicine. It is a member of the Daisy/Aster Family. It grows in high meadows, coniferous forests, and the western mountains at elevations from 3500 to 10,000 feet. It is native to western North American from Alaska to California and New Mexico, and east to Michigan. It is relatively easy to cultivate in the garden.

Identification: Arnica is a rhizomatous perennial growing from one or more erect stems. It grows between 12 and 20 inches (30 cm to 50 cm) tall.

The stems are hairy with two to four pairs of heart-shaped to arrowhead-shaped leaves. Cordate leaves

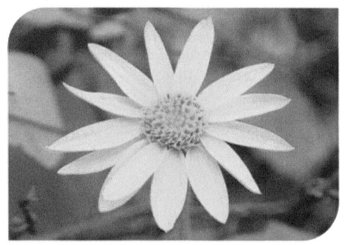
Arnica cordifolia, Pellaea, CC by 2.0

are often produced on separate short shoots, are coarsely toothed and wither when the plant flowers. The leaves on the upper part of the plant are hairy, like the stalk. Lower leaves have rounded tips. The flowers are small and yellow, forming 1 to 5 daisy-like flowering heads per plant, and each flower head has a golden yellow disc with 10 to 15 yellow rays. The rays are pointed and about 1 inch (2.5 cm) long. The entire flower head is about 2 1/2 inches (3.7 cm) in diameter. The seeds form in a small, hairy achene, about 1/2-inch (1.25 cm)-long. Flowers appear from May to August.

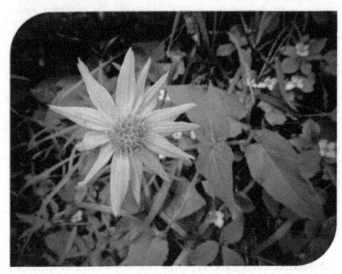

Heartleaf Arnica, Walter Siegmund, CC by SA 3.0

Medicinal Use: Use the flowers externally to reduce inflammation, reduce bruising, and for pain. It is antimicrobial and antiseptic. It can be used in small doses internally with great care.

How to Use Arnica on Skin: I often use Arnica externally on the skin as a salve or oil to promote healing in sprains, muscle pulls, contusions, and bruises. Use a diluted oil or salve on areas that need tissue stimulation and healing. Arnica treats common skin problems like infections, itching, and eczema.

Arthritis: Arnica is excellent at relieving arthritis pain, especially in cold weather. It warms the area and stimulates blood flow, and is anti-inflammatory. Rub arnica salve into the painful joint, or apply it as a poultice of bruised leaves or flowers.

Frostbite and Chilblains: Because it is warming and stimulates blood flow to an area, Arnica is used for the treatment of frostbite and chilblains. Use a poultice of leaves or flowers, or a salve or oil made with Arnica.

Bruises, Black Eyes, Muscle Aches, Inflammation, Sprains, Phlebitis, Carpal Tunnel, and Swelling: Arnica applied topically is useful in the treatment of a wide variety of external conditions. It reduces inflammation, warms the skin and muscle, relieves pain, and promotes healing. It is excellent for any strains, sprains, swellings, carpal tunnel, muscle soreness, and to reduce bruising.

Sore Throat and Toothache: For a sore throat or a toothache, try chewing the root. If the mouth is too sore for chewing, mash it and apply it to the swollen area. Gargling Arnica Tea is also effective for some people.

Other Uses of Arnica: Some people use Arnica to make homemade cigarettes, known as mountain tobacco.

Harvesting: When harvesting from the wild, pick flowers sparingly, never harvest rhizomes or roots; this destroys the plant. The plant will grow back as long as the rhizome survives in place.

I prefer the flowers for medicinal use but leaves and stems also contain beneficial properties. Pick flowers in the early afternoon, after the morning dew has evaporated.

Warning: Arnica can be highly toxic if taken internally. I do not recommend internal use, except homeopathically.

Avoid using undiluted Arnica preparations topically on open wounds, as it can cause inflammation and irritation. Dilute the oil and extracts with a carrier solution or oil if using on broken skin.

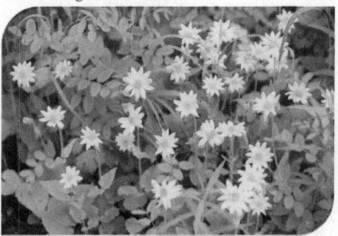

Arrowleaf Balsamroot, *Balsamorhiza sagittata*

Arrowleaf balsamroot, also known locally as the Oregon Sunflower, is a tough plant. It grows in grasslands, steppe, and scrubland areas, often on hillsides, in the western part of North America. It is in the Aster/Sunflower/Daisy Family.

Identification: Arrowleaf Balsamroot grows 1 to 2 feet (0.3 to 0.6 meters) tall. Its basal silver-green leaves grow up to 2 feet (0.6 meters) long and are arrow-shaped. Larger leaves are at the base of the plant and the leaves get smaller toward the top of the stem. Leaves are "wooly" and covered in fine white hairs.

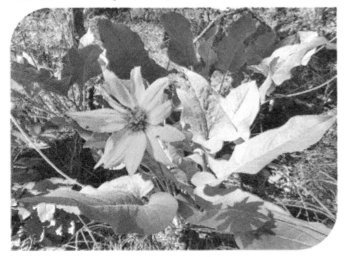

Flower stems grow from the root crown to 6 to 30 inches (15 cm to 75 cm) tall. Each flower stem has one flower head that resembles a sunflower with 8 to 25 yellow rays surrounding a disc. This plant grows from a deep taproot reaching 8 feet (2.4 meters) into the ground. It also has deep lateral roots that extend up to 3 feet (0.9 meters) around the plant.

Edible Use: This plant is an excellent food source. Its leaves can be eaten raw or cooked. Peel the stems before eating to get rid of the tough exterior. The seeds are nutritious and can be roasted like sunflower seeds. The root is eaten steamed or can be dried and pounded into a flour. The root can also be used as a coffee substitute.

Medicinal Use: The leaves, stems and roots contain medicinally active compounds. It acts internally as a disinfectant and expectorant.

Stimulates the Immune System: Taken internally, arrowleaf balsamroot roots enhance the action of the immune system, works as an antimicrobial, and stimulates the activity of white blood cells.

Toothaches, Sore Mouths, and Body Aches: Traditionally used to treat toothache pain and sore mouths by chewing on the root. Inhaling root smoke is said to treat body aches.

Sore Throat, Bronchial Congestion, Coughs, and TB: Balsamroot Tincture made from the dried or fresh root treats sore throats and loosens phlegm. Try putting your tincture into warm water and drink as a tea. You can also make cough syrup by simmering the root in raw honey (recipe below). Chew on the root to ease sore throat pain. Root infusions are used traditionally to treat tuberculosis and whooping cough.

Soothes Skin Burns, Wounds, Eczema, and Bruises: Use the balsamroot leaves as a compress on the skin to relieve pain and help heal burns, wounds, bruises, and rashes. Dry and powder the leaves or bruise and mash fresh leaves and place them on the skin or infuse them in oil for a salve.

Fungal Infections, Ringworm, Jock Itch, and Athlete's Foot: Use the dried and powdered root as an antifungal to heal common fungal infections. Apply the powder and leave in place to heal ringworm, jock itch, and athlete's foot.

Stomach Problems: The root, leaves, and stems are soothing for the digestive tract. Try a tea made from the entire plant.

Harvesting: Leaves and stems are easily harvested by cutting the stem and leaf from the plant. The root is more difficult because there is a very deep taproot as

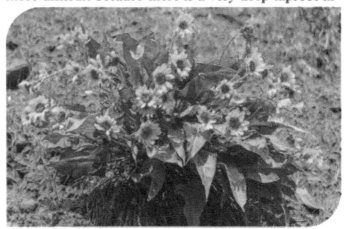

well as lateral roots and it often grows in rocky soil. Harvest the root in mid-spring to mid-August. You'll probably need to dig out a large area to get most of the root. Bring good tools and only take what you need from this slow-growing plant.

Recipes. Balsamroot and Raw Honey Cough Syrup: You'll need 3 to 4 Tablespoons of fresh Arrowleaf Balsamroot root, chopped into small pieces, and 1 cup raw honey. Bring the honey to a simmer and add the chopped balsamroot. Keep the heat at a low simmer for 2 to 3 hours. Strain the warm honey to remove the root pieces. Place in a clean jar and label and date. Use 1 to 2 teaspoons every 2 to 4 hours or as needed.

Bearberry, *Arctostaphylos uva ursi*, or *Arbutus uva ursi*

Also called kinnikinnik, uva ursi, hog cranberry, mountain cranberry, upland cranberry, bear's grape, and red bearberry, this herb is a small evergreen shrub that grows in northern North America and in higher elevations throughout the Appalachian Mountains. It likes acidic dry soils, especially sandy and gravel rich soils. It is in the Ericaceae (Heath) Family. It is commonly used in smoking mixtures.

Identification: The alternate paddle-shaped leaves are small and shiny with a thick, stiff feel. The underside is lighter in color than the green topside. Leaves are up to an inch (2.5 cm) long and have rounded tips. The leaves are evergreen, changing from dark green to

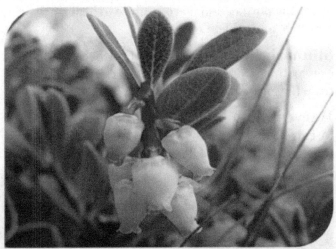

Bearberry, Jesse Taylor - Own work, CC by SA 3.0

a reddish-green and then to purple in autumn. The small dark brown buds have three scales.

Bearberry has small white or pink, urn-shaped flowers that appear in terminal clusters from May to June. They mature into pink to bright red fleshy drupes. The fruit is 1/4 to 1/2 inch (0.75 cm to 1.25 cm) in diameter and can remain on the plant until winter. Each mealy fruit contains up to five tiny hard seeds.

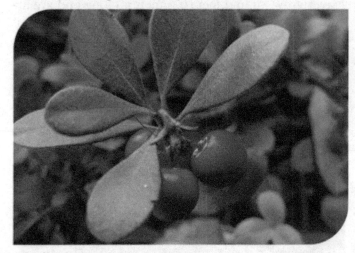

Bearberry Flowers, By Yvonne Zimmermann - Own work, CC BY-SA 3.0

The root system has a fibrous main root with buried stems that give rise to the stems of the herb. These trailing stems form layered mats with small roots and have stems growing up 6 inches (15 cm) tall when mature, with a reddish-brown bark. Younger branches are white to pale green.

Edible Use: Bearberry fruits are edible, but they are not tasty, so they are rarely eaten or used in cooking. They are sometimes used in pemmican.

Medicinal Use: The leaves and berries are used for medicine. I usually use it in tincture form for internal use.

Urinary Tract Infections, Nephritis, Kidney Stones, Cystitis, and Gout: Bearberry leaves treat kidney (nephritis), bladder (cystitis), and urinary tract infections extremely well. It is a diuretic, increasing the urine volume, and it has antiseptic properties that reduce bacteria populations in the kidneys, bladder, and urinary tract. It relieves bladder inflammation and helps relieves the pain of kidney

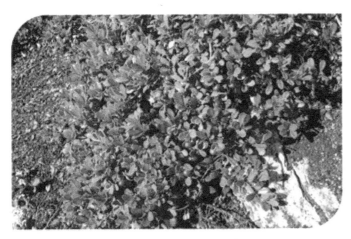

Bearberry, Walter Siegmund - Own work, CC by 2.5

stones. It also reduces uric acid in the body, and thus is useful in treating gout.

Bearberry leaves work best for urinary tract problems when the urine is less acidic or even slightly alkaline. Use at the first sign of infection. I often use it for UTIs as a blended tincture with Usnea, Goldenrod, and Oregon Grape Root, and also drink unsweetened cranberry juice or take a concentrated cranberry supplement. To decrease acidity, follow a vegetable-based diet, eliminating meat and milk products from the diet until the problem is eliminated.

Painful Sex in Women and the Urinogenital System: Bearberry tea or tincture treats long-term inflammation of the urethra in women. The tannins in the berries and leaves have a strong astringent action and reduce inflammation in the urinogenital system.

Vaginal Infections: Bearberry is an effective internal treatment against vaginal infections, including yeast infections. It has astringent and anti-inflammatory effects that help soothe the vaginal region. You can also use the leaf and berry tea as a douche or sitz bath twice a day.

Post-Partum Use and Uterine Hemorrhage: Drinking Bearberry Tea soon after giving birth helps increase uterine contractions and prevents

hemorrhages. It helps prevent post-partum infections and helps incisions heal. It can also be used as a douche or sitz bath due to its astringent and tightening effects. Not for longer-term internal use if the mother is breast-feeding.

Prevents Scurvy: Bearberry berries and leaves are rich in vitamin C, which is necessary to prevent Scurvy. In winter months it can be difficult to find adequate sources of vitamin C. Drinking bearberry tea or eating its berries adds vitamin C to the diet.

Stomach and Intestinal Cramping: Bearberry has muscle relaxant properties that soothe stomach and intestinal cramping. It also has antiseptic properties that are effective against the most common causes of diarrhea and stomach upsets.

Harvesting: Bearberry leaves can be picked from mid-spring to mid-autumn. Pick the mature berries before the first frost.

Warning: Bearberry should not be used by people with high blood pressure, by pregnant women, or women who are nursing. Bearberry can induce nausea in some people and can cause stomach irritation. Soaking the bearberry leaves overnight before use may help. Not for continued long term use. Best used for acute treatment.

Recipes. Bearberry Leaf and Berry Tea: *Soaking the leaves and berries before brewing the tea removes some of the tannins and helps reduce digestive discomfort if using internally. You can also use the leaf only.

3 Tablespoons of dried leaves and berries, chopped, 1-quart (1 Liter) water. Soak the dried leaves and berries in cold water overnight or for up to one day. Drain. Bring a quart (liter) of water to a boil. Add dried leaves and berries. Reduce the heat to a simmer and cover tightly. Simmer the tea for about five minutes. Turn off the heat. Allow the tea to steep, tightly covered for 30 minutes. Strain. Drink one cup, two to three times daily, lukewarm on an empty stomach.

Bee Balm, Oswego Tea, *Monarda didyma*

Bee Balm is also known as Oswego Tea, horse mint, Indian nettle, Red Bergamot and Scarlet Bergamot. It gets the name Oswego tea because of its use by the Oswego Tribe. It is in the Lamiaceae (Mint) Family and is easily cultivated in the garden. This is a great herb to plant to attract hummingbirds, bees, and butterflies. It is a perennial and grows naturally in much of North America, Europe, and Asia.

Identification: Bee balm has straight, ridged, square stems and grows to 3 feet (0.9 meters) tall. Its course opposite leaves can be smooth or have a thin coating of fine hairs. The leaves have a strong fragrance and are 3 to 6 inches (7.5 cm to 15 cm) long. Their showy flowers range in color from deep pink to bright red to purple. They are approximately 1 ½ inches (3.75 cm) long and are grouped in dense heads of many flowers. They bloom in mid to late summer. The plant spreads on underground shoots, increasing the size of the plant every autumn. The plant in the center will begin to die back after three to four years.

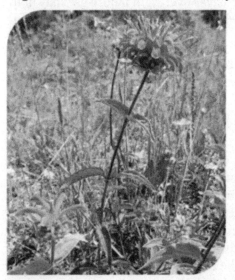

Edible Use: Oswego tea is made from dried leaves of the bee balm plant. The leaves and flowers are edible. Bee balm flowers are lovely as a garnish in salads, and dried leaves can be used like sage to flavor meats.

Medicinal Use: Leaves and flowers are used medicinally.

Menstrual Problems: Bee balm is an anti-spasmodic, and large doses of bee balm tea cause the uterus to contract, bringing on the menstrual period. However, it can also cause miscarriage and thus should be avoided during pregnancy

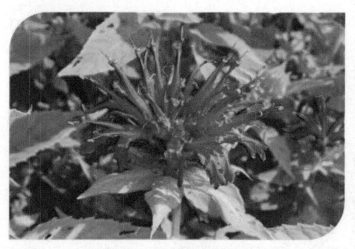

H. Zell, own work, CC 3.0

Colds, Sore Throats, and Congestion: Bee balm leaves are useful for treating colds, sore throats, and nasal and chest congestion in the form of a tea or in a steam vaporizer. Breathe in the vapors to open sinuses and clear congestion from the lungs.

Fevers: Oswego/Bee Balm tea is a mild diuretic, expelling water from the body through both sweat and urination. Sweating helps cool the body and reduce fevers.

Nausea, Vomiting, Flatulence, and Stomach Problems: Like most mints, bee balm has a soothing effect on the stomach and can calm flatulence, nausea, and vomiting. However, it is not appropriate for use with nausea caused by pregnancy. Large doses can cause miscarriage.

Nervine for Calm: Bee balm works similarly to Lemon Balm as a nervine, though it is less powerful than Lemon Balm for this use.

Stings, Scrapes, and Rashes: Bee balm is wonderful in a healing salve and helps soothe bites, stings, and rashes.

Harvesting: Pick the leaves in the mid to late morning after the morning dew has dried. Pick your yearly supply during the summer and dry them for future use. Collect the flowers when they are beginning to fully open. Dry them and store them in a sealed jar in a dark place.

Recipes. Oswego Tea: You'll need 1 teaspoon Oswego Tea/Bee Balm Leaves and 1 cup boiling water. Pour the boiling water over the tea leaves and allow the tea to steep for 5 to 10 minutes. Strain out the leaves and drink.

Black Cohosh,
Actaea racemosa

I find black cohosh to be a very valuable herb for menopause, and I rarely use it for other uses, except as a supplementary herb. It balances hormones, which helps many conditions without curing them. Black cohosh is in the Ranunculaceae (Buttercup) Family. Black cohosh is native to eastern North America. It is found as far south as Georgia and west to Missouri/Arkansas and the Great Lakes region. It grows wild in small woodland openings.

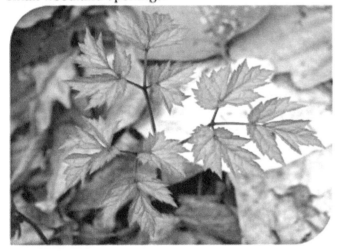

Identification: Black cohosh is a perennial with large compound leaves that grow from its rhizome. It grows up to 2 feet (0.6m) in height with distinctive serrated basal leaves that can be 3 feet (0.9m) long, growing in sets of 3 leaflets. Flowers bloom from June to September on an 8-foot tall stem, with racemes (flower clusters) up to 20 inches (50 cm) long. These white flowers occur in tight clusters with a white stigma surrounded by long stamens.

The flowers have no petals or sepals. A distinguishing feature is the sweet, putrid smell of the flowers that attracts flies, gnats, and beetles. The fruit is a 1/4-inch to 1/2-inch (0.74 cm to 1.25 cm) long dry follicle containing several seeds.

Medicinal Use: I mainly use black cohosh root for menstrual problems and menopause, although it is also useful for digestive problems and as a sedative. The best benefits are achieved when black cohosh is taken regularly long-term. Often it takes a month or more before benefits are noticed. The root is used medicinally.

Menopause, Menstrual Problems, Improved Ovulation, and PCOS: Black Cohosh works to balance hormones in women, helping to relieve menopausal symptoms such as hot flashes, moodiness, night sweats, headaches, heart palpitations, vaginal dryness, and mental fog.

It is also used for menstrual problems, painful intercourse, decreased sex drive, and Polycystic Ovary Syndrome (PCOS) and has been shown to improve ovulation in women.

Osteoporosis: By balancing hormones, black cohosh reduces bone loss caused by osteoporosis in women.

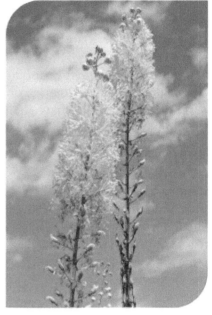
Black Cohosh Inflorescence, H. Zell, CC by SA 3.0

Reducing Anxiety and Aiding Sleep: Black cohosh has a sedative effect that calms the nervous system and reduces anxiety. It promotes restful sleep.

Digestive Problems: For digestive problems, crush a small piece of black cohosh root and boil it in a small amount of water. Drink the water to relieve stomach pain and intestinal problems. It helps improve digestion and elimination and prevents gastric ulcers. Black cohosh is only moderately effective for other digestive problems. There are better remedies out there.

Warning: People who are allergic to aspirin, have liver problems, have issues with seizures, or have a high risk of blood clots or stroke should not use black cohosh.

Pregnant and breastfeeding women, women with endometriosis, uterine cancer, or breast cancer should not take black cohosh.

Bleeding Heart, *Dicentra formosa*

Bleeding heart is a calming herb and is useful for the nervous system after a shock or an accident. It is also known as Pacific Bleeding Heart and Western Bleeding Heart. It is in the Papaveraceae (Poppy) Family and grows in moist areas of coniferous forests in the Pacific Northwest.

Identification: Bleeding heart is a perennial with fern-like, lacy, divided leaves. It grows from a rhizome and reaches 18 to 24 inches (45 cm to 60 cm) tall when mature. Heart-shaped dangling pink flowers bloom in clusters from mid-spring through autumn. Flower stems reach above the leaves, each with 5 to 15 blooms. Seeds form in pointed, pea-like pods. Depending on the weather, the plant may go dormant during the hot summer months. They have shallow rhizomes that are easy to harvest but are also sensitive to foot traffic.

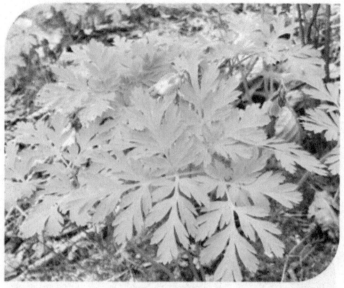

Medicinal

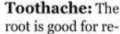

Use: Use bleeding-heart with great care and in small doses as it is a very potent narcotic and is toxic in higher doses. The root is mostly used, though the flowers and leaves also have medicinal properties.

Toothache: The root is good for relieving toothache pain. Chew the root and place it on the painful tooth.

Bruises, Sprains, Joint Pain, Nerve Pain: A compress made with Bleeding Heart Decoction or by heating root pieces in water and applying them as a poultice is effective in relieving nerve and muscle pain and helping bruises and sprains to heal.

Shocks to the Nervous System, Anxiety, and Nervous Disorders: Bleeding heart root decoction and tincture are both effective in relieving anxiety and nerves. It is effective in calming people after a shock, loss, or trauma. The plant has sedative and narcotic properties.

Muscle Tremors: Compounds in bleeding heart are calming and relaxing for the nervous system. They relax the muscles and suppress muscle tremors exhibited in some nervous system disorders.

Diuretic: This diuretic herb helps flush toxins and other poisons from the blood, liver, and kidneys. However, there are safer herbs for this use.

Increases Metabolism and Stimulates Appetite: Bleeding heart calms the nervous system while increasing the metabolic process, often giving you more energy and an increased appetite.

Cancer and Swollen Lymph Nodes: Bleeding heart tincture has been used traditionally for the treatment of cancer, swollen lymph nodes, and enlarged glands.

Harvesting: Bleeding heart is a rare plant and is becoming endangered in some areas. Check the status in your area before collecting and do not overharvest. Use it sparingly because it is rare in the wild, or, even better, grow your own supply so that you do not disturb the plants growing in the wild. Gather the roots of bleeding heart in the summer, if the plant goes dormant, or in the autumn when the leaves begin to change and after the seed pods have matured.

Warning: Avoid using bleeding heart during pregnancy or breast-feeding. Use bleeding heart sparingly, a little goes a long way. Do not use if you have liver disease. Do not use in combinations with other sedatives and note that it can cause a false positive for opiate use on a drug test. Consult a medical professional before use.

Recipes. Bleeding Heart Tincture: Finely chopped fresh or dried bleeding-heart rhizome to fill ½ a jar, 80 proof or better alcohol such as vodka or brandy.

Place the rhizome pieces into a clean jar with a tight-fitting lid. Cover the herb completely, filling the jar with alcohol. Cap and label and place it in a cool, dark cupboard. Shake the jar daily for 6 to 8 weeks while the tincture steeps. Strain, label, and store. Usual dosage is 10 to 20 drops of fresh tincture, and 15 to 30 drops if using dried roots. Use with care.

Bloodroot, *Sanguinaria canadensis*

Bloodroot is mainly for the treatment of skin cancers, ulcers, and wounds that won't heal. I have always known the herb as bloodroot, but it is also called red-root and red puccoon.

The juice is red and quickly dyes the skin and has been used by the Algonquin Tribe to paint the skin for ritual. It is in the Papaveraceae (Poppy) Family.

Use with great caution! This herb grows in eastern North America in moist thickets and dry woods and on floodplains and near streams.

Identification: Bloodroot is a stemless, rhizomatous wildflower that blooms in early spring. The herb grows from 6 to 10 inches (15 cm to 25 cm) tall. The leaves go dormant in mid to late summer. When the bloodroot flower is sprouting, it's usually wrapped by one deeply-scalloped, grayish-green, palmate basal leaf. Bloodroot has a hermaphroditic flower that has 8

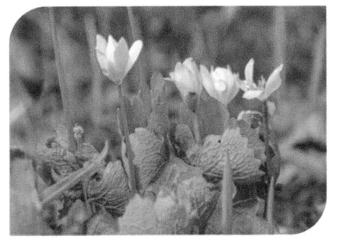

to 12 fragile white petals, yellow stamens, and two sepals positioned below the leaves, which fall off after the flowers open. The root is a blood-red rhizome that will branch out and grow new rhizomes.

Medicinal Use: Caution is advised. Bloodroot is a toxic plant, and serious problems can arise. Use small doses only as advised by a medical professional or find an alternative plant. The root is used medicinally.

Skin Cancers, Ulcers, Moles, Skin Tags, Warts, Eczema and Other Skin Conditions: Treating skin problems is what bloodroot does best. However, use with great caution and in moderate amounts as it will also kill healthy cells and can cause permanent scarring and sloughing of the skin. Traditionally, people made and applied a salve from bloodroot to the affected area.

They covered it with a bandage and left it in place for a week or so. Usually, only one application is required, but extensive areas, deep lesions, or other tough cases may require repeated application.

The bloodroot kills the cancerous or damaged cells and covers the area with a scab.

Leave it alone to heal, and check the area to be sure that all of the cancer is removed so that it doesn't

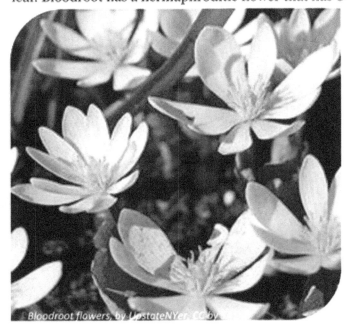
Bloodroot flowers, by UpstateNYer. CC by

return. The bloodroot also has anti-inflammatory, anti-bacterial, anti-fungal, and anesthetic properties that help the skin to heal while relieving pain. The salve can be used to remove skin tags, warts, moles and other unwanted skin lesions. Apply the salve directly to the lesion, keeping it well away from the healthy skin. If you decide to use this plant do so with great caution and in small doses. I use a facial mask once a month with a very small amount of bloodroot in it (along with other ingredients). This is a good example of my utilizing it in small and infrequent doses.

Treating Respiratory Problems: Bloodroot is a bronchial muscle relaxant used to treat asthma, whooping cough, influenza, and as a treatment for croup.

Gastrointestinal Problems: Bloodroot powder treats gastrointestinal bleeding, abdominal cramps, nausea, and vomiting. In large doses, it acts as an emetic, causing the very problems it treats. Use with great care or find an alternative herb.

Diphtheria, Tuberculosis, and Respiratory Illnesses: Small doses of bloodroot decoction are an antibacterial agent useful for the treatment of bacterial diseases such as diphtheria, tuberculosis, asthma, bronchitis, and pneumonia. For respiratory illnesses, it has the added benefit of cleaning out the mucus and congestion and suppressing coughs. However, I prefer other, safer remedies. For sore throats, you can dilute the decoction in a glass of water and use it as a gargle.

Menstrual Problems: Small doses of Bloodroot Decoction are beneficial for treating menstrual problems including excessive bleeding and cramping. Again, I prefer other plants for this purpose.

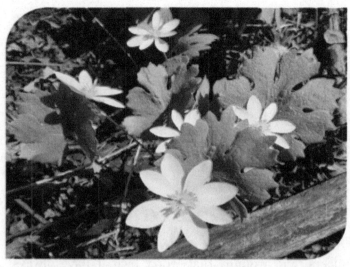

Dental Care: Extracts from bloodroot help fight infections like gingivitis and prevent the formation cavities, tartar, and plaque. Add a drop of bloodroot decoction to your toothpaste for this purpose or use a diluted tea as a rinse.

Harvesting: Wear protective gloves to protect your hands from staining red and to avoid the medicine being absorbed through your skin. Best harvested in autumn when the strength of the plant is returning to the root and the tops are dying back. Dig up the root and the surrounding area, removing the rhizomes. Leave a few behind for next year's plants. Dry for future use.

Warning: Great caution is advised. Bloodroot is a toxic plant that can cause tunnel vision, nausea, and death. Do not use bloodroot if you may be pregnant or if you are nursing. It may also cause permanent scarring or disfiguration when used topically.

Blue Cohosh, *Caulophyllum thalictroides*

Blue cohosh is also known as squaw root or papoose root for its use to induce labor. It is a perennial member of the Berberidaceae (Barberry) Family.

Do not confuse it with Black Cohosh. They are very different. It is found on the floor of hardwood forests in eastern North America. It prefers moist soil, hillsides, and shady locations with rich soil.

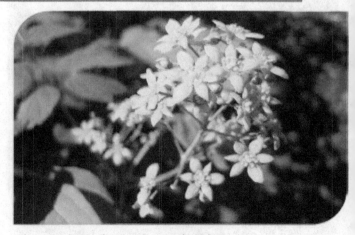

Blue Cohosh, Biosthmors - Own work, CC by SA 4.0

Identification: A single smooth stalk, 1 to 3 feet (0.3m to 0.9m) tall, grows from the rhizome, and contains a single three-lobed leaf and a fruiting stalk. Its leaflets are serrated at the tip and the leaves turn a bluish-green hue when mature. It has deep blue fruits.

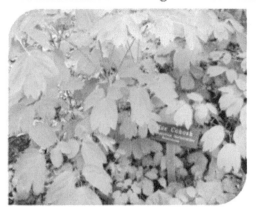

Blue Cohosh, by Carol, CC by SA 3.0

Medicinal Use. Childbirth: The root has oxytocic properties that promote childbirth. Do not take during pregnancy until 1 to 2 weeks before the due date and only under a doctor's care. It causes powerful uterine contractions that are regular and productive, encouraging a quick and easy birth. It also has a calming effect, helping the mother relax between contractions and reducing pain.

Menstrual Problems: Blue cohosh root is used for menstrual problems, including delayed menstruation, cramping, and profuse hemorrhage.

Harvesting: Harvest blue cohosh root in late autumn, when it stores its strength. You can also harvest the rhizomes in the spring, just as the new growth begins, if needed. Dry and store the roots for future use.

Warning: Do not use during pregnancy. Do not use for estrogen-sensitive diseases such as endometriosis, fibroids, and certain cancers. Blue cohosh can elevate blood pressure so careful using for heart patients and people with high blood pressure. Excessive dosage can cause nausea, vomiting, and a lack of muscle coordination.

Butterbur, Arctic Sweet Coltsfoot, *Petasites frigidus*

Butterbur, or Sweet Coltsfoot, is a plant that grows in moist areas throughout the Northern Hemisphere. The name butterbur reportedly came about because the leaves were used to wrap butter for keeping. It is also called bog rhubarb. It is in the Aster/Daisy Family. Note that Arrowleaf coltsfoot (*P. frigidus* var. *sagittatus*) has the same medicinal properties as butterbur; it has arrow-shaped leaves.

Butterbur or Sweet Coltsfoot is not the same plant as *Tussilago farfara*, known commonly as coltsfoot and also in this book, though they are closely related.

Identification: Butterbur or sweet coltsfoot flowers appear in February and March, before the larger basal leaves that arrive in late spring. The flowers have a sweet scent, and are often the first flowers seen in the new year in the cold wetlands in the North. A cluster of white to purple-pink flower heads appears on the tip of a fleshy stalk, which is covered with sheathed leaves.

The flowers give way to silver-white seed heads and its large basal, rhubarb-like leaves arise near the flowering stalk directly from an underground rhizome. The basal leaves are palmately divided and their underside is "wooly" with white hairs.

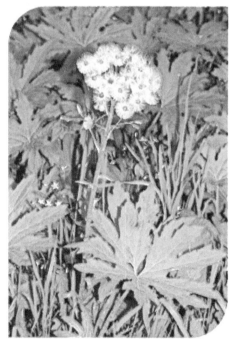

Petasites frigidus by Walter Siegmund (talk), Own work, CC-BY-SA-3.0

Edible Use: The flowers, flower stalks, and leaf stalks are edible in limited amounts when cooked.

The ash (after burning the aerial part) is a good salt substitute.

Medicinal Use: The roots, mature leaves, and stems are all used medicinally. It is antispasmodic, anti-inflammatory, a vasodilator, and mucilaginous. I use it as a tea or a tincture. Only collect mature leaves, as young leaves contain small amounts of pyrrolizidine alkaloids, which are hepatotoxic.

Allergies: Butterbur leaf is very effective for allergies, including hay fever, reducing histamine and leukotriene release. It has been shown to be as effective as many prescription allergy medications without causing drowsiness.

Bronchial Spasms, Chronic Coughs, and Spasmodic Airways and Asthma: Butterbur leaf is useful against asthma and restricted bronchial passages. It reduces the sensitivity and the frequency of attacks. As an antispasmodic, it reduces spasms of the bronchial tract while also relieving inflammation, and is excellent for any chronic cough like those caused by emphysema or bronchitis.

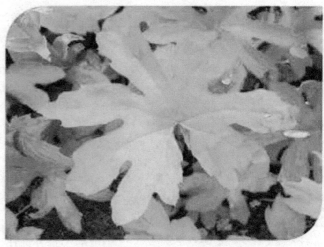

Petasites frigidus by Stan Shebs, Own work, CC-BY-SA-2.5

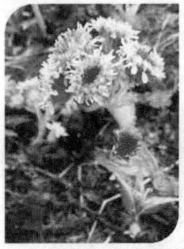

Migraine Headaches: The herb relaxes vasoconstriction and relieves inflammation that can trigger migraine headaches. Like feverfew, it is best taken daily as a preventative rather than as a rescue treatment, though it works as a cure as well. I often pair it with Feverfew in tincture form. Taken daily, butterbur leaf reduces the incidents of migraines.

Inflammation and Muscle Sprains: The plant is a strong anti-inflammatory and antispasmodic. Externally a root poultice can be used to treat inflammation and pain due to a muscle sprain or strain.

Harvesting: Harvest roots in spring. Harvest the leaves and stems throughout the summer once they are fully grown. Young leaves contain small amounts of pyrrolizidine alkaloids, which are hepatotoxic.

Warning: Avoid using butterbur if you have liver problems. Do not use if you are pregnant or breastfeeding, or for children under age 7. Adverse reactions can include GI symptoms, nausea, flatulence, and gassy stomach. Allergies are possible.

California Buckwheat, *Eriogonum fasciculatum*

California Buckwheat is in the Polygonaceae (Buckwheat) Family. It is a wild buckwheat species and is commonly known as eastern Mojave buckwheat. This shrub is a native to the Southwestern United States and Northwestern Mexico. It grows on dry slopes, canyons, and washes in scrubland and coastal areas.

Identification: *Eriogonum fasciculatum* is varied in appearance. Sometimes it is a compact bramble and sometimes it is a spreading bush approaching 6 feet (1.8m) in height and 10 feet (3.0m) wide. It has numerous flexible slim branches.

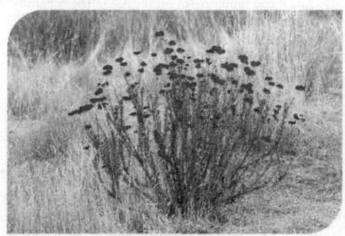

California Buckwheat, Stan Shebs, CC by SA 3.0

Its leaves and are 1 1/2 to 2 inches (3.75 cm to 5 cm) long and less than 1/2 inch (1.25 cm) wide. Leaves grow in a whorled cluster at nodes along the branches. They are wooly and leathery on the undersides and roll under along the edges.

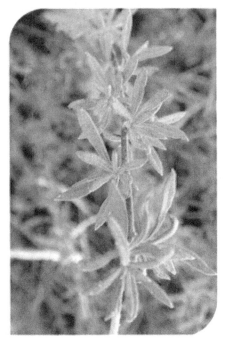

Its flowers are dense clusters that are 1 to 6 inches wide (2.5 cm to 15 cm). Each distinct flower is white and pink and only a few millimeters across. It blooms from May to October. It has light brown small seeds.

Edible Use: The seeds are eaten raw or dried for later use. Seeds can be ground into a powder and used as a flour. Young sprouts can also be consumed, and the seeds can be sprouted to eat.

Medicinal Use: The seeds, leaves, flowers, and roots are all used for medicine. Older, mature plants are more potent. The roots are dried and ground for medicine and a strong, thick tea is made from the leaves or the roots.

Wound Care: The leaves, flowers, and roots are used for skin wounds. Fresh leaves or flowers can be applied as a poultice. Ground leaves and ground roots are mixed with water or oil and applied as a poultice. California Buckwheat Tea can be used as a wash.

Colds, Coughs, and Sore Throats: A mild leaf tea works for colds, coughs, and sore throats. The hot root tea can also be used for colds and laryngitis.

Diarrhea and Stomach Illnesses: For diarrhea and other stomach troubles, use a strong decoction made from the roots of California Buckwheat. It cleans out the system and gets rid of irritants.

Oral Care: For sore gums or for use as a mouthwash, use a weak leaf tea. It is a mild pain reliever and calms inflammation. Swish a mouthful of tea around for a few minutes, then spit it out.

Headaches: For headaches and other aches and pains, use a strong tea made from the leaves. It relieves the immediate pain and flushes toxins from the system.

Heart Health: A tea made from dried flowers or dried roots helps prevent heart problems.

Harvesting: The seeds mature in early autumn and dry right on the plant. Wait until the seed pods have dried and turned to a rusty brown before harvesting. Once dried, they can easily be hand-stripped from the plants into open tubs or bags. Harvest older roots as they contain more medicine.

Recipes. Strong California Buckwheat Root Tea: 1 tablespoon California buckwheat shredded root, 1 pint (500 ml) of water. Mix the root into the water and bring to a boil. Reduce the heat to a simmer. Cover and simmer the tea for 15 minutes.* Strain and serve warm or cold. *For a weaker tea, reduce the brewing time to 5 minutes

California Buckwheat Leaf Tea. 1 teaspoon California buckwheat leaves, dried or 1 tablespoon fresh, 1 cup boiling water. Pour the boiling water over the leaves and steep for 5 to 10 minutes. Strain.

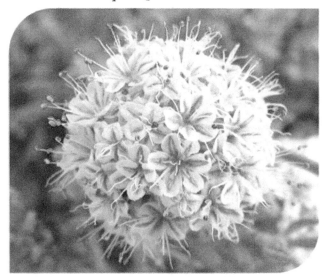

Cardinal Flower, *Lobelia cardinalis*

Cardinal flower is a beautiful showy plant with brilliant red flowers. This plant is hard to miss. It is in the Campanulaceae (Bellflower) Family. It grows in wet soil, swamps, stream banks, and along rivers.

Identification: The flowers are a cardinal red color and are 2-lipped with five deep lobes. They grow on an erect raceme approximately 2 to 3 feet (0.6m to 0.9m) tall and flower during the summer and autumn. The toothed lanceolate to oval leaves grow 8 inches (20 cm) long and 2 inches (5 cm) wide.

Medicinal Use: Traditional uses for cardinal flower are below. It isn't used as often as it used to be in herbal medicine but is still an important plant to know. All parts are used medicinally.

Bronchitis: Cardinal flower is used as an expectorant for bronchitis.

Epilepsy, Diphtheria, Tonsillitis: The anti-inflammatory and narcotic properties of the roots help it treat convulsive and inflammatory diseases such as these. It relaxes spasms and allows the body to heal.

Eye Diseases: A weak tea made from 1 teaspoon of root or leaves per cup of boiling water is useful as an eye wash.

Sprains, Bruises, and Skin Irritations: As an external application for relieving pain and encouraging healing in sprains, strains, bruises, and other surface irritations, try Cardinal Flower tea or a Lobelia Seed

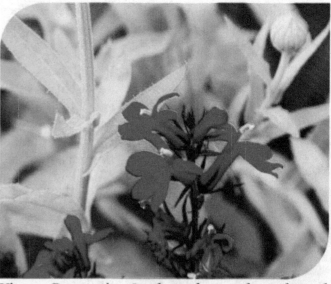

Vinegar Preparation. It relaxes the muscles and speeds healing though I do prefer other plants for this use.

Warning: Some other plants in the *Lobelia* genus are toxic, so it is wise to be careful in the use of cardinal flower since it could potentially be toxic in larger doses. Symptoms of toxicity would include nausea, vomiting, diarrhea, excessive saliva, weakness, dilation of pupils, convulsions or coma.

Lobelia Vinegar Preparation: Use the fast method only in emergencies. A slower maceration is best. Ingredients: 4 ounces (113g) powdered Lobelia seed and 1-quart (1 Liter) of vinegar. Macerate the vinegar and seed powder for seven days, shaking daily. Filter mixture through a coffee filter to remove the seed powder. Store in a cool, dry place. Fast Method: Place the vinegar and seed powder in the top of a double boiler and cover. Bring water to a simmer in the lower pot. Warm the vinegar mixture this way for 1 hour. Cool and strain.

Cat's Claw, *Uncaria tomentosa*

Cat's Claw, or uña de gato, grows in Central and South America, where it grows profusely in the rainforest. The root and vine bark are imported here for medicinal use. It is a useful plant and I try to keep a supply on hand. It is in the Rubiaceae (Bedstraw/Madder) Family.

Identification: Cat's claw, *Uncaria tomentosa*, is a tropical woody vine whose hooked claw-shaped thorns give it its name. The vine grows to a length of up to 100 feet (30meters), climbing anything in its path.

The bright green elongated leaves grow in opposing pairs. They have a smooth edge that may be rounded or come to a point. The flowers are yellow, trumpet shaped, and have five petals. The barbs are hook-shaped and curled like a cat's claw.

Medicinal Use: The inner bark of the vine or root is used. It is taken as a powder, in capsules, as a tea, or as a double-extracted tincture.

Cancer Treatment and Prevention: Cat's claw prevents and helps treat cancer. It contains anti-inflammatory, anti-oxidant, and anti-tumor properties that prevent cancer cells from developing in the body. It helps the immune system fight existing cancerous cells by enhancing white blood cell function. People in chemotherapy report that it helps relieve pain and other symptoms related to chemotherapy drugs.

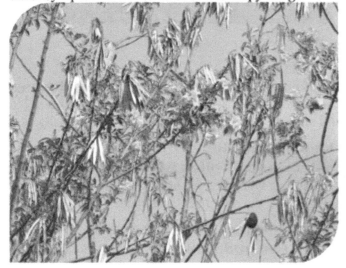

Irritable Bowel Syndrome, Crohn's Disease, Colitis, Ulcers, and Other Gastrointestinal Issues: Cat's Claw helps support the digestive system, relieving inflammation in the stomach and intestines. It has anti-bacterial, anti-fungal, and anti-viral properties that help rid the body of the underlying causes. It fights diseases of the intestines, stomach, and liver while restoring the body's natural flora and healing the digestive system.

Anti-Inflammatory and Autoimmune Conditions: Inflammation is a cause of many body diseases, including autoimmune diseases, arthritis, and heart disease. Reducing swelling in joints, wounds, and bodily organs helps the body heal faster and reduces pain. They are still researching its use in certain autoimmune diseases, and some recommend not taking it if you have an autoimmune issue due to the way it boosts the immune system.

Osteoarthritis and Rheumatoid Arthritis: The anti-inflammatory effects of this herb are very beneficial for osteoarthritis and rheumatoid arthritis. It calms the inflammation, reduces swelling, and relieves the associated pain.

Powerful Anti-Viral: Cat's claw is useful in treating viral diseases due to its quinovic acid glycosides. It is used to treat herpes, Epstein-Barr, hepatitis B and C, HPV, HIV, Dengue Fever, and other viral diseases. I would try it against any of the tropical viral diseases, given the need.

Helps the Body Heal, Chronic Fatigue Syndrome: Its anti-inflammatory and anti-bacterial properties help the body from getting an infection and calm the body's response to the damage, helping it heal. It also helps people with Chronic Fatigue Syndrome.

Lowers Blood Pressure: Cat's claw increases circulation throughout the body and helps lower blood pressure for people with hypertension.

Supports the Immune System and Help for Mold Exposure: Cat's claw contains isopteropodin, which helps increase the body's white blood cell count, eliminates free radicals from the body, and helps fight infection. Its anti-inflammatory and anti-oxidant properties also help with mycotoxin exposure.

Regulates Female Hormones and the Menstrual Cycle: Cat's Claw helps regulate the female hormones that keep the menstrual cycle regular and helps to alleviate bloating, cramping, and mood changes that are associated with it. If you are pregnant or trying to conceive avoid this plant. It can cause miscarriages and may prevent conception.

Detoxification: Cat's claw is beneficial in detoxifying the whole body and cleansing the blood and lymph. It is excellent at removing toxins, drugs, heavy metals, and other foreign substances from the body. It also boosts the effectiveness of the kidneys, spleen, pancreas, and digestive system due to its cleansing effects.

Warning: Do not take cat's claw if you are pregnant, nursing, or trying to get pregnant. Do not take if you have an autoimmune disorder. It may cause a flare-up. Consult your health professional if you are taking blood thinners or any other prescription drugs as it interacts with some of them. Side effects can include nausea, diarrhea, and dizziness.

Cleavers/Bedstraw, *Galium aparine*

Cleavers, also called Bedstraw, catchweed, sticky weed, and goosegrass, is an annual plant that grows in damp, rich soils along riverbanks and fence lines in eastern and western North America and is found worldwide. It is in the Rubiaceae (Bedstraw) Family. You often find the plant and its seeds stuck to your clothing like Velcro after walking through it.

Identification: A climbing hairy, almost sticky, stem grows from a thin taproot to a height of 2 to 6 feet (0.6m to 1.8m). The plant has coarse leaves with a variable shape. The leaves grow in whorls around the stem, and the stem, leaves, and fruit are usually covered with small, spiny hairs. Its leaves may be oblong to lance-like or even linear. Cleavers flowers are small and white or greenish-white in color and flower from early summer until autumn. The flowers have a sweet smell.

Edible Use: Cleavers are edible. I prefer them cooked as their hairs and hooks get stuck in my throat when I eat them raw. Their seeds can be roasted as a coffee substitute. They are a good green to juice and drink.

Medicinal Use: Cleavers are astringent, anti-inflammatory, diuretic, detoxifying, febrifuge and promote sweating. It is effective both internally and externally. I use the leaves for medicine and infuse them cold into oil, water, or a tincture. Do not boil.

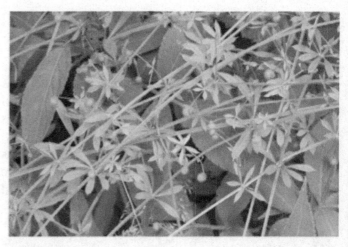

2 Cleavers growing over the tops of other plants, Mike Pennington, CC by SA 2.0

Rejuvenate the Skin, Slow the Signs of Aging: Cleaver tea is said to have a toning effect to tighten skin and smooth out wrinkles when applied externally.

Detoxify the Body, Drain the Lymphatic System, and Swollen Glands: Cleavers are a diuretic. They work well to remove toxins from the body and to clean the lymphatic system.

Skin Disorders, Acne, Psoriasis, Eczema, Abscesses, and Boils: Cleavers works internally and externally to improve the condition of the skin, detoxify the blood and lymph, and reduce inflammation associated with these conditions. They are also antibacterial, which helps treat the underlying infections. Use both internally and externally for these conditions.

Kidney Stones, Bladder and Urinary Tract Infections: Cleavers are very effective at treating bladder infections, urinary tract infections, and kidney stones. It dissolves stones, clears obstructions, and flushes them out of the body. The antibacterial action is effective at curing the underlying infections.

Cancer: Research has been done that supports the use of cleavers to treat tumors, especially those of the breast, skin, head, neck, bladder, cervix, prostate, and lymphatic system.

Chickenpox, Measles, and Fevers: To treat chickenpox and the measles, try cleavers internally to treat the disease and externally on the skin to relieve the itching and general discomfort from the rash. Cleavers also helps bring down the accompanying fever.

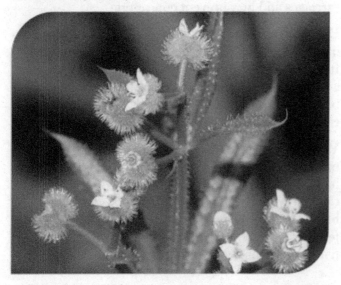

3 Cleavers flowers and fruit, Alvesgaspar, CC by 3.0

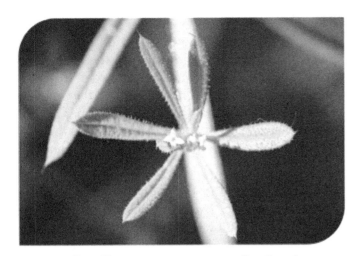

Stop Bleeding, Burns, and Sunburns: Freshly picked cleavers leaves are excellent for stopping bleeding in wounds, cuts, or other surface bleeding. Apply the leaves directly to the wound. It also reduces inflammation and speeds healing. The leaves can be made into a poultice for larger wounds.

Tonsillitis, Sore Throat, Glandular Fever, and Prostate Problems: Cleaver juice works well for glandular problems like tonsillitis, glandular fever, and for prostate problems and prostate cancers. When fresh juice is not available an infusion can be used, although it is not usually as effective as the juice for these issues.

Harvesting: Harvest cleavers in spring to mid-summer and use fresh or dry for later use.

Recipes. Cleaver Juice. Fresh cleavers leaves and water. Wash the fresh leaves thoroughly and place them in a blender with a small amount of water. Use only as much water as needed to blend. Blend the leaves into a pulp and strain out the juice with a fine sieve. I recommend making a large batch of juice and freezing the extra. Most people drink 2 cups daily to treat cancers and tumors.

Club Moss, *Lycopodium clavatum*

Club moss is a vascular spore-bearing plant and propogates via spores. It is in the Club Moss Family, Lycopodiaceae, and is not a true moss but is more closely related to ferns and horsetail. Club Moss is found worldwide and is also called staghorn, ground pine, and running pine,

Identification: The yellow-green leaves are scale-like and short and taper to a fine feathery point. The 3 to 4-foot-long, ground-hugging stem of this plant is highly branched with small, spirally arranged scaly leaves. The stem runs along the ground producing roots at frequent intervals. It resembles the seedling of coniferous trees, though there is no relationship between them. Its spores grow on two or sometimes three yellow-green barrel-shaped cones that are on small, 6-inch (15 cm) stalks.

Medicinal Use: Mostly the spores are used in medicine, but sometimes an extract of the entire plant is used.

Respiratory Problems: Club moss spore decoctions are used to treat ailments like chronic lung, bronchial disorders, and other respiratory issues.

Congestion, Colds, and Flu: Club moss spores act to dry out mucous membranes and relieve congestion. Try a 1/4 teaspoon of the spores mixed into a glass of water three times a day until the congestion clears.

Urinary Tract Disorders: Club moss is a diuretic, increasing the amount of urine expelled and flushing toxins from the body. To treat urinary tract problems, use a decoction of the whole plant. Common usage is 1 to 2 tablespoons of the decoction 3 to 4 times a day.

Skin Conditions: Club moss spores treat many different skin conditions, including allergic reactions, sunburns, psoriasis, eczema, fungal infections, chickenpox, contact dermatitis, hives, and insect bites and stings. Make a salve with the spores of club

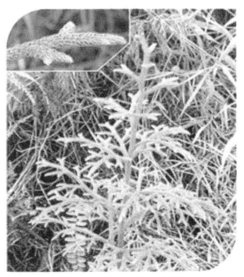

moss. The spores can also be applied lightly as a

powder and rubbed into wounds, folds of skin, or anywhere that you prefer not to use oil. The powder absorbs moisture and helps heal wounds.

Rheumatoid Arthritis: A decoction of the entire plant is said to help rheumatoid arthritis symptoms.

Flatulence: Both constipation and flatulence can be treated with spores from club moss. As little as 1/4 teaspoon mixed with water eases symptoms and resolves the problem.

Kidney Diseases: Club Moss Decoction made from the whole plant is used to treat kidney disease and related disorders. It works to eliminate kidney stones and cleanse the system.

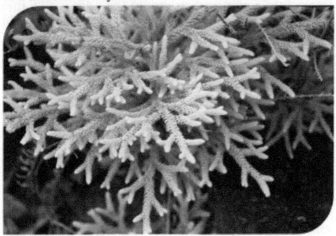

Wound Treatment: Open wounds and sores that refuse to heal are well served by the application of club moss spores. Apply the spores as a powder and rub it into the affected area.

Harvesting: Harvesting of club moss should be done when the spore heads are dry, mature, and ripened, though the spores can also be harvested while still green. For a ripe plant just cut off the plant and spread them on a sheet to dry until the cones open. Shake them and collect the spore powder. To collect the spore heads from green cones, cut off the cones and break them open. Place the cones in a paper bag and place them in a cool, dry place to open. When the cones open, shake out the spores and remove the remaining plant material.

Warning: Club moss contains small amounts of alkaloids, which are a toxic substance and can cause paralysis to the motor nerves if consumed in large amounts.

Recipes. Club Moss Decoction: 1 ounce of ground or finely chopped club moss plant, 2 cups of water. Bring the water to a boil and add the club moss plant. Turn the heat down to a slow simmer and simmer the decoction for 15 minutes. Allow the decoction to cool and strain out the herb. Keep the decoction in the refrigerator and use within 3 days. Use a maximum of one cup daily, split into 4 or more doses.

Club Moss Salve. 5 ounces (150ml) of organic olive oil or other carrier oil, 1 ounce (28g) of shaved beeswax, 1 tablespoon of club moss spore powder. Heat the olive oil gently over very low heat in a double boiler. Add the club moss spore powder. Keep the oil on very low heat for 20 to 30 minutes while the spores release their medicine into the oil. Add the shaved beeswax and stir until the salve is thoroughly mixed. Do not strain out the spores. Pour the salve into a sanitized jar and cover it tightly. Keep the salve refrigerated if in a very hot climate. Apply 2 to 3 times daily, as needed.

Coltsfoot, *Tussilago farfara*

Coltsfoot is in the Aster/Daisy Family, and is closely related to Butterbur. It is native to Eurasia but has naturalized in the US and Canada. It is also known as coughwort, podbel, and son-before-the-father.

Identification: Coltsfoot is a rather unusual perennial. The flowers look like dandelion, but they appear early, in April, and die before the leaves appear. It grows between 4 and 6 inches (10 cm to 15 cm) tall and is usually found in open areas with disturbed soil.

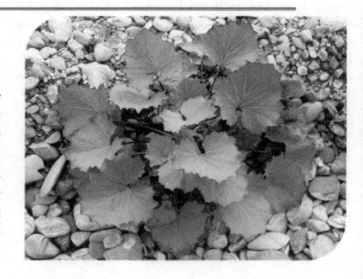

Made in the USA
Las Vegas, NV
07 June 2024

90840316R00083